A Healing Initiation

A Healing Initiation

Recognise the Healer Within

by Melissa Hocking

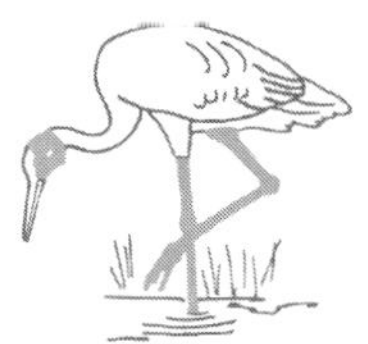

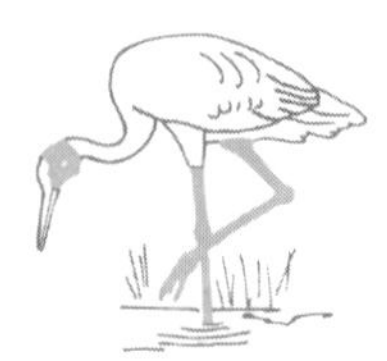

Published by Brolga Publishing Pty Ltd
ABN 46 063 962 443
PO Box 12544, A'Beckett Street, Melbourne, Victoria, Australia, 8006

email: sales@brolgapublishing.com.au
web: www.brolgapublishing.com.au

The information in this book is neither diagnosing nor treating any specific health challenges. It is sold with the understanding that the authors and publishers are not engaged in rendering medical, health, or any other kind of personal professional services in the book The reader is responsible for seeing to and continuing any medical treatment and care as advised by their own medical, health or other competent professionals. The author makes no claims, promises or guarantees. All material in this publication is for informational use only, and put forward to assist the individual in their personal development. Use of this material is the responsibility of the reader.

National Library of Australia
Cataloguing-in-Publication entry

Hocking, Melissa Ann, 1972- .
A healing initiation : recognise the healer within.

ISBN 9781920785963.

ISBN 1 920785 96 5.

1. Spiritual healing. 2. Mental healing. 3. Self-care, Health. 4. Alternative medicine. I. Title.

615.852

Printed in Singapore
Cover Design by David Khan
Typeset by Amy Gibbs

For my greatest guides,
My most patient and indulgent teachers,

Jack,
Colby
and Teagan

contents

Part Five: What will you do with this?

Part Six: Your Journey

Appendices

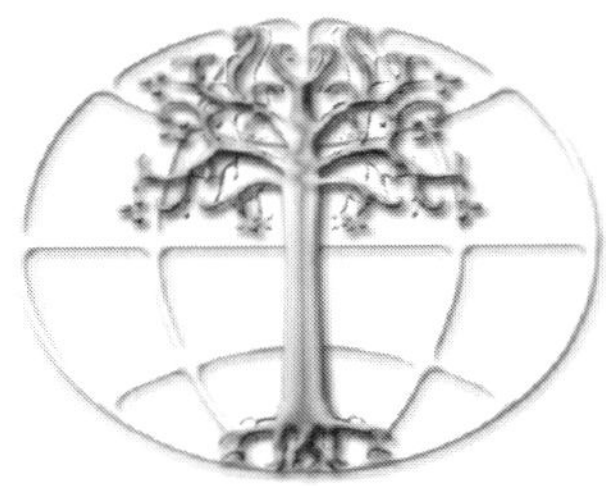

acknowledgements

"Guard within yourself that treasure, kindness. Know how to give without hesitation, how to lose without regret, how to acquire without meanness... Know how to replace in your heart, by the happiness of those you love, the happiness that may be wanting in yourself."
George Sand (Amandine Dupin) 1804-1876

From me to you: I thank you...

This work is the result of years of research and a personal quest to share this with all who can use it (*everyone*). Both of which, the quest and the research, continue. As I continue to work with clients, to teach, to speak and share, and now write, the work does continue to evolve. After all, *Ancora Imparo.*

I've been privileged to be guided by the teaching and wisdom imparted from a number of great teachers, mentors, scholars, scientists, medical professionals, and generally great people, collectively friends, and above all else they own my gratitude. Many you will find quoted throughout this volume. All of these people come to the team recognising the importance of this work, and the ability we each have to use it. Their input is truly quantum: timeless and immeasurable.

What a desperately confusing and lonely road this would be without them!

My gratitude to you:

Jack, Colby, and Teagan, my personal in-house university, each of you housing unique and unbridled wisdom. I am in the privileged role of calling you all "my children", when so often I feel like yours. I have no words that are adequate for the enormity I feel for each of you. I love you.

Andrew Hocking, now my "former" husband, and always one of my greatest friends and allies. Test subject for all the written lessons, sounding board for all the input (no mean feat, I tell you), and my great "partner in parenting". One whose wit far outstrips any other, whose warmth and generosity is always welcome, I thank you.

Chris Warren, my soul brother, my true friend, my beloved ally in the trenches. Your truth inspires my own, your courage I lend as often I can, your hand in mine as we go forward I appreciate above all else.

Libby Strugnell. This incredible and powerful work we are doing with children would not be happening without you. Should my courage falter, your absolute knowledge steps in. I know that my gratitude doesn't need to be spoken to you, but the world should know of your extraordinary beauty, gentleness and the powerful gift that is you, Lib. You bring wisdom to the future… you bring the children.

Helen Carter, my former business manager, and beloved friend, who left us with extraordinary speed under the guise of lung cancer (*great endorsement Helen!*). Her belief and the power she brought to the early stages of opening this up for people was nothing short of phenomenal. In my memory I still hear you, in my heart I still feel you… all the same, wish you were here.

Savannah Woods, my exceptional editor, aka GG (my Gift and Guide), true to her contract, to her purpose and always to her friend. I adore walking this planet beside you, GG. Your friendship and support is cherished intensely. Love you.

Kate Brede, Meg MacFadyen, and Helen Libby, beside me they are the legends in lesson. Thank god for email! I learn so much from and through you. I love you guys. Even more, I love laughing with you. Namaste.

Larry Macy, with the loyalty of a labrador and the courage of a lion, my wonderful, inspirational friend. Your support is treasured.

My adopted grandparents, Aunty Ze and Uncle Bill. Quiet nights in the stifling heat of the living room, reading and sharing the books that we read… you were and are my sanctuary. I admire you for so many reasons: Your absolutely unconditional love and patience, always seeing the beauty within first and your strength when you took on an extraordinarily strong child. You never caved, and I respect you above all others for it.

Thank you. Thank you. Every day I aspire to be as beautiful as Aunty Ze.

Two Bears, offering to me that day in the canyon one of the most prominent and important lessons in this life. I hold true to my promise, my friend and adopted "Indian father": I will continue to "Walk my path. And walk it True.".

Of the great teachers, mentors, scholars, scientists, medical professionals, and generally great people, collectively friends, I also thank Lynn Mewburn, Scott Alexander King, Tanja Fairweather, Graeme Evans, David Locke, Sonia Russian-Thomas, Dave and Jane Lale, Leanne Synan, Eric Pearl, Janine Shepherd, Ayesha Hilton, Paul Ribet.

To my publisher, the team at Brolga, hand selected for its integrity, my thanks. And especially to Mark Zocchi, a man of honour, truth and strength. Mark, in a world where integrity struggles to find its feet, you stand solid. Your role in this is no small role. Thank you, my friend.

To all the clients that have come to my door, my gratitude for allowing me to share in your personal miracle is the utmost privilege.

To the ill, disabled, the injured and heart broken, thank you for sharing lesson with me.

To those that attend the courses and choose to share this work, you are so much more powerful than you know. The ripples are going out, and the choices you are making, make the difference.

To the exquisite children that flow in and out of my door, such blessing all should experience. Thank you little empowered warriors.

To all those who would oppose, belittle or attempt to quash me in any way, I thank you for the strength and resilience that keeps me moving forward. And for fuelling the challenge to bring this forward.

To my family

Linda (*sister extraordinaire*) I could not do this without you. Reece (*number one naysayer*), beloved brother-in-law. And Moos (*Madeline*) who lights up the world all on her own, and tears up the road as she does it. Miss Maddy Moo, "Arnmahs" loves you.

Uncle Barry and Aunty Pat, The Hocking Clan, and all the raucous relatives. Oh c'mon, you know you're all "raucous". Ta.

Mum. I love you.

To Dad. Bye Dad. Keep the veranda step warm until I get Home.

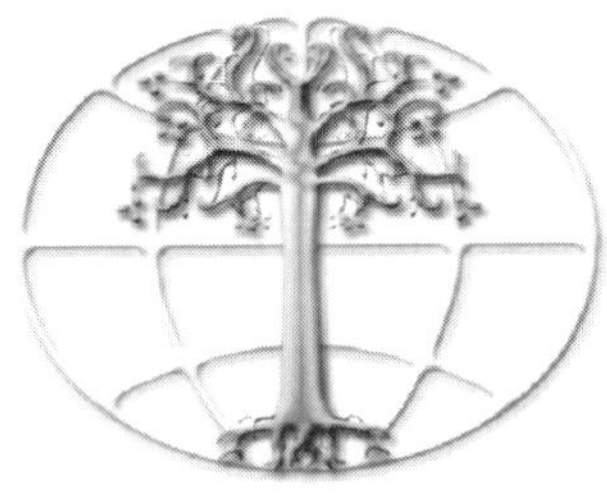

Preface

Ancora Imparo.

The interpretation for this Italian phrase is "I am still learning". Originally I came upon this phrase during officer training in the Australian Army, a rich educational environment to say the least. These days "Ancora Imparo" has become my motto in this life and on this journey. And I love that the education and knowledge is never ending nor stagnant, and that I am more "pioneer" than "professor".

If you're thinking that I've started this book with a disclaimer, perhaps you're right. My personal, plaguing peeve in life is pretence, (a lesson in tolerance I am still learning), and so I would rather share this motto, than suggest that I have all the answers. If this book ended up all of 27 pages, then I would have called it a "brochure" and passed it on, rather than load another two hundred pages with filler.

Years ago, accidentally attending the wrong lecture, I crossed a certain line and entered into an astonishing adventure in healing. The path that has led to the discovery of the **Quantum BioEnergetic balancing technique**™: a process of healing truly unprecedented in our time.

Quantum based frequencies are enabling healing as never before. The results are extraordinary. And already, as you're reading, ***you*** have the ability to use this. For yourself, and if you so choose, for others.

I extend an invitation to you: to experience healing as never before.

For you can and will do so, as you venture forth into this book.

One of the most difficult decisions for me in putting this healing process to paper was how and when to start. Where do you start writing when the work itself is constantly evolving and changing? How do you describe this "thing" in simple, understandable and usable terms? Over the last couple of years, as I have been pushed, prodded, encouraged and nagged to get on with writing this, I would try to explain the complexities of the energy and the changes I'd seen occurring only recently, and say "How can I explain what isn't finished yet?" All sorts of people were putting their two cents worth in. As a guest at a clairvoyant circle I was to discover that even channelled entities were getting in on the act!

Finally, a great friend took me into a warm embrace and said gently, "Mel, just put down the basics. That way people can start where they need to." He then went on to give me the titles of my next three books after this one! Clearly he has a plan! But for now, let's get *you* started…

I truly appreciate the time you're taking to experience and learn more about you. That's really what this is about; finding ***your*** way with the immense gift of healing. Never underestimate that this is ***your gift***. For most of you, it may not be your "primary" gift, but instead an accelerant as you travel toward whatever unique and extraordinary gift is yours. These frequencies are amazing like that…

I've often said it, and I'll apologise now because no doubt, I will repeat myself to you, but the physical healing is often the least of this. I wonder if these frequencies showed themselves initially in a healing capacity so that we, shackled by humanity, bound by our duality in consciousness, would be able to accept them at a rudimentary level. Over the years, seeing many clients, my experience has shown me so, so much more. There's a whole encyclopaedia to transcribe in this discussion alone!

So, welcome to the next step on your journey. It is my privilege to be a part of it. Clearly all I can offer you is my own perspective, and really that is all it is.

This is your journey.
Take what you need,
Discard what you don't,
and, please, be gentle with me.

All the best,

Melissa Hocking

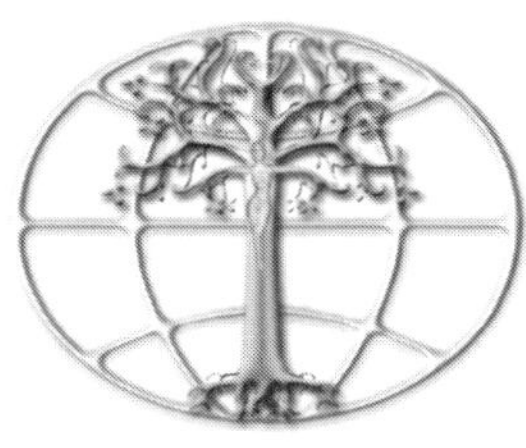

Initiation

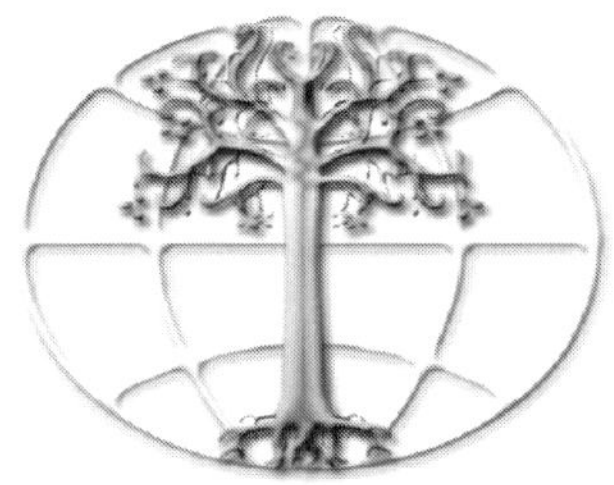

Introduction

You see things; and you say, 'Why?'
But I dream things that never were; and I say, "Why not?"
George Bernard Shaw
"Back to Methuselah" (1921), part 1, act 1

The Crack of the Starter's pistol

"Yep, uh-huh, it's a tumour." The doctor was groping about my lower abdomen with incredible indifference, in the way only a doctor could.

"Yep, already the size of a golf ball." He stood up staring absently at my abdomen. "Well," he sighed, "we'll have to take care of that, won't we." Then he turned and called to his receptionist to take some notes for him.

I was 19 years old. Just finished High School, and started a scholarship at University in Engineering, which I already knew I despised. Nineteen years old, just starting out with my whole life ahead of me; alone, frightened and bewildered by what was happening around me.

The receptionist walks in.

The doctor continues his indifferent monologue, as the fog closes in on my brain. "Yes, Judy, she has three tumours, roughly the size of golf balls in her uterus…", *Tumours? You only hear the word "tumour" when you hear about…*

The doctor's voice returned to my ears in time for me to hear, "...feel they are cancerous. Yes." He finally met my eyes, "You will need to see an oncologist."

Standing up to leave, he added a few cursory instructions to the receptionist. In that moment I found my voice.

"Cancer? I have cancer?"

He stopped in the doorway and looked at me blankly, his eyebrows curiously raised, apparently surprised that I was still there, "Yes," he said and walked out.

As I look back now, had my hearing not been shrouded within the horror of such diagnosis, no doubt I would have heard the crack of a starter pistol; for this was the moment when I crossed the starting line, journeying into the very role I now live. The direct route leading me to this purposeful life started with that diagnosis.

Already a lot had happened in my life, a chaotic cacophony of events prior to this diagnosis. All had happened to create who I had become. Yet this was the moment, when the "contract", the task I was here to fulfil, came into play. I put foot upon the pathway to here, a pathway of unprecedented healing.

I use quantum based frequencies to trigger living bodies to heal themselves.

Yes, I do. And so can you.

The best thing about this enormous gift, is that right now, as you sit there reading, you already have it within you to use these amazing frequencies.

Yes, this amazing healing ability is yours. You can use this for yourself, for your dying tomatoes, for your arthritic pussy cat, or, if you so choose, you can help other humans. Myself,

I do all of the above.

This process of healing is a non-invasive, hands-off form of healing whereby a body is immersed within quantum based frequencies and is then able to instigate and facilitate an appropriate healing for itself.

This process of healing is the **Quantum Bioenergetic Balancing Technique**™.

I am not the "healer". You'll find as much as possible I refrain from calling myself "healer", although it has been difficult in the process of writing this book to find another term! So forgive me if, for convenience, I use the term "healer". I do work with energy healing (although I'm not altogether comfortable with "energy" either), and I am certainly not the designer of it all.

I am an instrument, a vehicle through which these frequencies can be implemented and applied. It is my privileged role to immerse a body within these frequencies, and watch as that body prioritises what it needs to heal, and then heals itself. Immersed within these frequencies, living bodies are enabled to recognize healing codes that until recently were residing dormant within, and activate them.

The clientele that walk into my rooms suffer from any number of permanent disabilities, chronic illnesses and terminal disease. I have worked on individuals of all ages from babies in-utero, to my oldest client to date who as I write she is about to turn one hundred. And every day, I watch in wonder as I have the privilege of both facilitating and witnessing the most incredible healings.

Above all, what has become most obvious is that such ailments are no longer "permanent", "chronic", or "terminal". Our biology has evolved, as has, its ability to heal itself! We are able to heal ourselves, and in many cases, the healing happens in an instant.

When I say "living bodies", I mean *all* living bodies, human of course, but also plant, and animal, fish, even water.

I have not yet seen a living body that *does not react* to quantum bioenergetics. Sure, there are people who do not receive the healing *they* anticipated, but always there is a healing of some design. The simplest explanation I can give you is that the body itself had a greater recognition of the healing priority, than that which the client consciously deemed pertinent. Instead the body responds exactly as is appropriate, at the time, for them. A plan uniquely designed for that individual.

With these pages, I have the immense privilege of giving to you the amazing gift you have within, a blessed discovery that is to say the least significant in the evolution of healing. To be able to hand this to you, was always the intent for this gift. And as such it is an essential element in the evolution of both the frequencies, and the human. Perhaps you should read that sentence again, for it is no small matter, the evolution of the human.

What I am not doing is presenting you with something brand new and exciting that nobody else knows about. I'm not that special, I'm afraid. Even the concept itself is not "new". Research and proven results in frequency therapy date back centuries.

What has been recently discovered and introduced to us is this readily available *quantum based* frequency.

What I am going to share with *you* is the innate, already present gift you have to utilise this incredible healing ability. Through the role I am in everyday, as a Healing Facilitator, I'm going to assist you in recognising this, for as I said, the knowledge is already within you.

As you're reading, perhaps you are already feeling something activating within. Something deep inside has started to dawn, your awareness of this gift is stirring. You may suddenly become very "aware" of your hands, or at least a new sensation in and/or around you that is strong enough to draw your attention.

How? As you are reading, you too are discovering, just as

I did. Your journey of discovery, chaperoned by yours truly, is actually a journey of recognition. Your own biology is remembering, your energy anatomy ascending... Can you believe it? You're already doing this! There will be more to follow.

To date there are numerous writings, ranging from New Age authors, to Scientists, to volumes of Scripture, that have predicted, or attempted to explain, the changes in the planet, in the Human and in the code within us. And there will be many more to follow. The Dead Sea Scrolls themselves, their format being more a documentation, are an adventure in explanation with much yet to show us. Change has indeed occurred, and continues to do so, on many levels. Time has indeed sped up. (No, it's not just that it feels that way now that you're getting older. It has truly sped up.) Magnetic North is on the move. There is a distinct change in the energy as it exists on the planet. A good internet search engine can readily access and verify all of this information for you, and more.

What is truly enormous in these exceptional changes is that ultimately in all of us it all comes back to a single living body. In fact back to a single, living cell, and within the cell the framework or "matrix" that holds this ancient code. Great spiritual leaders, scholars, scientists, medical practitioners, are collaboratively investigating and researching the evidentiary directives we have been given toward self rejuvenation from and at the cellular level.

With the energy of the planet shifting and affecting all things, it should be expected that the Human Body would also shift. After all, few people still believe that the human is an autonomous entity. We are aware more now than ever before, that there is a balance that occurs, a symbiotic affect, between all things: planet, nature, human, and a greater power, albeit God, (the Universe, Spirit, Higher Self, Life, whichever term you feel comfortable with).

These changes, palpable and evident across the globe,

inevitably affect all that are related upon this planet. Even us. Just by acknowledging this, you've increased your knowledge and your potency as a healer both of self and others. Changes are now able to occur within that single body, yours and others, that weren't available to us only a short time ago.

These frequencies are old. In what way they are "old" I don't really know, nor would I guess, but it is clear that they have been almost "lying in wait". When a body is first exposed to these frequencies there is moment of "recognition", where that body struggles for a moment to remember how to let them flow, how to make it fit, get comfortable with it, how to accept this shift and ultimately to use it. When you're working on someone utilising these frequencies, it's quite a distinct feeling beneath your hands as that recognition occurs, and that body starts to flow.

That recognition suggests a memory within, rather than a dawning from without.; as if we had the ability to transfer these frequencies at the dawn of time, but not the recognition or ability to know how they were to be utilized – with disuse perhaps they atrophied and only now as we have grown and evolved have we taken the next step in our human evolution. Now with our recognition of and education about quantum bioenergetics, we are able to use our innate abilities at the cellular level. With this change we're now able to recognize an extraordinary healing ability that until recently we were unable to comprehend or to access.

It raises the question of whether these frequencies are creating a new DNA "fingerprint" within us, as some have theorised. Or as it has also been suggested, a case of dormant DNA is being roused, the very "junk" as science once referred to it, activated. But this "recognition" raises the question if, in fact, DNA's role is far more *communicative* than constructive. The recent international collaborative studies of the human genome have shown "gaps" in the DNA matrix that are suggestive of cellular memory.

As to the question of exactly *how* the healings occu. indulge me in my technical answer;

I'll get back to you on that.

What is it that is imprinted within a living physical body that recognises a priority, a need for healing? Is it memory or knowledge we were born with or just plain luck? To the last I can say "no". I can make you this promise; I won't pretend to know the answers, either. I can tell you that I have given intent for the answers to come forth, and they are. But in this, your introduction to your own amazing gift, I will show you what I do know, what we are discovering and venture to discover and even a few theories, so you too can take this forward.

In recent times the use of terms such as "DNA" and "cellular" have been used prominently in all sorts of environments. Global marketing groups are utilising these terms to enhance sales of any number of products. And you know, when a term becomes a marketable asset, it has a common value in the marketplace, and hence becomes common place in the minds of the people. Amid this new awareness, the human consciousness, on all levels has started to address DNA and the genome, cell structure, and human biological reaction beyond known medicine. Globally the population is seeking "wellness" as never before. The timing of this is not an accident.

Our knowledge of DNA, similar to our knowledge of the brain, is still in its infancy. As only we would, the DNA we couldn't readily identify, let alone understand, was clumped into a collective group known technically as "junk". Clearly something we're happier to write off as rubbish, than admit to our own lack of knowledge.

Globally scientists currently collaborating upon the human genome, now refer to that in-between as the "gaps". No longer is it "junk", as science has started to see, evidently, that these gaps hold the as yet discovered potential of the

;. In regard to the healing sessions through which
hat "in-between" that wears the greatest question
ow?"

The science in this healing process, as I write continues to have some significant holes in it, and for good reason. Pure science, as we know it, is not yet capable of understanding, or measuring what is occurring in these gaps, or for that matter, in these healings. Quantum frequencies and the measurement of an infinite number of outcomes is in our linear model of measurement, difficult to obtain. Of course research is underway, but we continue to hit a "gap" ourselves for there is still that as yet immeasurable "in-between".

That ego thing that defines us as humans and at the same time restricts us as humans, until recent decades, had restrained and hindered our scientific development on the whole. We viewed science in an almost backwards process! We took the facts that we had measured and "understood", and hypothesised upon them, rather than looking at the wonder of something, and asking how it came to be.

To paraphrase George Bernard Shaw

"Some look at what is and ask "Why?". Some look at what could be, and ask, "Why not?"

Rather than seeing the wonder before us and learning from it, until recent times we have been caught in the belief of an omnipotent existence, within our own conscious mind that made us obnoxious enough to believe we already knew what was relevant. And then, from that point, went on to anticipate relevant scientific findings.

Yet, it is that very history that now forces us to put that ego in our back pocket, and go forward with our vision a little less dogmatic. (Sadly, because really, it would have been far more comfortable to have stayed where we were, wouldn't it? You have to love that comfort zone.)

Once upon a time great prophets, scientists, and philosophers were punished, or even put to their deaths for their claims and discoveries. Throughout history, as time has gone on, they were proven to be right in their claims.

In more recent times awareness of a greater presence than merely us, ensures that we would take bolder, and not always mathematically justified, measures in moving forward in science. The last fifty to sixty years are evident in this.

And all of this stems back to a single individual body. At a cellular level and hence at an energetic level.

So already, this early into it, we've raised a number of questions in order to fill in the gaps, and on many levels; the science, the physical, and the spiritual. For now, let's bring it back to what we're here for…

Healing

Healing is a system of balance. Healers don't heal, they balance. It makes sense, doesn't it? After all, on such a brilliant scale, as we discussed before, required for our very existence, there has always been a required synergistic balance between primary elements; planet, human, spirit.

The individual biological reaction to a session, with a balanced healer, is what heals. Human biology itself is an exquisite sculpture in balance. It is the individual human reaction that heals, not the healer. Can you see the difference as to what we have chosen to believe for the longest time?

Over centuries we have sought a healing solution from source outside ourselves. We would feel a pain, or realize a loss in movement and seek out medicinal guidance or the assistance of someone we viewed to be more specialized than ourselves when it came to healing. The medical fraternity, through no real fault of their own for they too have learnt from history, has had a similar approach to healing, and perpetrated the continuing reliance on outside sources, rather than joining the innate abilities within the patient to the balancing abilities of the healer, be they medical, homeopathic or metaphysical.

When approaching a medical practitioner for an illness or injury, it was traditionally treated in the immediate state. You would be given pain relief for the level of pain you presented at the time, and appropriate medications to abate inflammation or infection as it had presented when you were there. And this treatment, for a large portion of us, has been adequate and indeed effective, so that the situation would not worsen, and your health could improve again. Indeed your body would be put into such a position that it could once again, balance itself. Such medical treatment has kept me alive doing just that; thankfully.

The true source of the health issue, what actually lead to the current situation, was rarely addressed in current Western medicine, and often considered irrelevant. Caught in our own wonder and, yes, a little of that omnipotent ego, western medicine lost focus on causative issues going beyond the purely physical.

Traditional Chinese medicine, (TCM) on the other hand, is one that recognizes the source cause when addressing the physical. A Chinese herbalist first explained to me the understanding that "when the heart is troubled, all other organs tremble". The effect of emotion, and hence the mind set of the individual, was an essential element in structuring treatment. Rarely in TCM are you prescribed treatment for a single issue, instead TCM practitioners work to balance the relevant system, and ultimately the entire physical system.

Again, balance. Healers don't heal, they balance. Whether it's your oncologist prescribing a stringent schedule of chemotherapy, your osteopath focussing on some cranial work, your surgeon removing your gall bladder, or me immersing you in quantum bioenergetics, all of us are working to achieve the same end: *To achieve an environment of balance within the body so it can then heal itself.*

Calling Western medicine's approach "backwards" is a

little unfair. Instead it's *immediate*, very much a Band-aid solution, as treatment is for the symptoms in the immediate situation. Our increasing need for instant gratification may have brought about this approach.

Perhaps Plato put it best, when he said, *"The great error of our day in the treatment of the human body is that physicians first separate the soul from the body."*

More and more I am seeing articles and papers written on the necessity for science to reunite with spiritual in order for that science to move forward. This isn't such a new concept. The answers are in fact bound within the tradition or the culture from whence it came.

The channelled entity, *Kryon*, tells us *"You can never separate the physical from the spiritual. Scientists have wanted to do that from the beginning. They actually pride themselves on the empiricism of their scientific method, and that it is completely separate from anything spiritual. The real joke is that at the heart of physics and biology is the spiritual plan of matter and life. It hides within the atomic structure, and also within the biology of each human."*

My own research, my own incidental education in this, appoints to a massive interconnecting matrix of the science and the spiritual in itself. True spirituality, being far beyond religion, meant that I sought out education from all genres. In the face of my own immense and incredible healings, restriction to traditional education would be almost blasphemous, and so I ventured into that which is labelled 'the new age'.

Sadly, Western medicine's growth now is also hindered greatly through fear of being sued. The general population has developed such a litigious nature that along the way, instead of simply denying our own responsibility, which is our usual approach, western culture found a way of actually putting it, legally, upon someone else! True shirking of responsibility on a soulful level!

A client came to me after having surgery for lung cancer,

seeking to aid his recovery. He sat down and told me how his GP had originally suspected cancer, and sent him to a particular hospital for assessment. After travelling some distance to get to the hospital, he undertook some tests, and they found nothing, so he returned home. Some weeks later, again his doctor referred him to the hospital, as he still was suspicious. This time the tests showed quite an advanced cancer. They scheduled him immediately for surgery, then treatment.

This gentleman was telling me this story because he'd just instigated legal action against the hospital for missing the cancer the first time!

He said to me, "It's disgusting, isn't it?" I replied "It certainly is! After all if they hadn't found it when they did, you'd be dead by now. Perhaps "gratitude" would suit you a little better than 'litigation?' His jaw dropped. And apparently he dropped his law suit almost as fast.

From my own perspective I see great and enormously positive changes occurring in Western medicine. More and more doctors are able to involve, if not embrace, other modes/methods and practitioners of healing. These days, I am asked into hospitals to work on patients. It's not officially prescribed treatment, and when they write it on the patients medical chart it is listed as "healing"(which must be terribly confusing for administrative staff!), but nonetheless its recommended "therapy" by their physician. If one medical professional is to introduce me to another, they tend to introduce me under the banner of "complimentary medicine". You have to like that.

Back in the old days, in my role as an Anatomical Physiologist, I ultimately ended working primarily in rehabilitation. Although recently, whilst lecturing at a course, I told the students "I used to work in rehabilitation, and now I work in…well, rehabilitation." My best description of an anatomical physiologist is a mechanical engineer for the human body. At the musculoskeletal level I would rebalance, reshape, and reintroduce function to the gross motor movement of a body. Various doctors and therapists would refer their patients to me for a more finely tuned approach to aid their recovery. I worked on all sorts of people from the elite athlete to personally training everyday people to simply lose a few pounds, and all sorts in-between. A fantastic job!

I was never actually taught any sort of methodical approach when assessing a client. When I earned my double degree it was tailored for me, so it wasn't a standard physiotherapy or medical training. It turned out that it was a huge asset to me as I entered this profession unencumbered by any existing methodical paradigms.

When a client came to me, I would look at them from the perspective of how the human body can be, and what we needed to change in the client's body in order for it to be as it should. I never doubted that any single body could recover from where it was. Even back then I would go right into the depths of research to create a plan, basically from the cell level up, and orchestrate an environment for that body to repair itself. (Not dissimilar to what I do now, right?).

Be under no illusion, this was not easy work for the clients but few ever complained. A gentleman came to me after having melanoma removed, with huge divots of flesh cut out of a major muscle group and barely able to walk due to the resulting overall weakness. Of course he was told there was no real hope of recovery, but he might be able to walk comfortably in time. 12 weeks later he was able to play football with his son again, and we went for a 3 kilometre run together.

Anyone that knows me will tell you that I have an inbuilt requirement for symmetry. It's *not* an obsession, but close to it (I can hear friends scoffing as I write.). Even my tattoo is symmetrical, and placed on my body in the most symmetrical place I could put it. So I couldn't resist, when rehabilitating someone, to rebalance them entirely. It wasn't a conscious decision as such; to me it just made sense that in order to maintain a working system, it needed to balance.

Usually when someone has a major illness or injury, the body naturally compensates in order to keep functioning. So I would find that a body had become hugely asymmetrical, musculoskeletally, as the clients gait had altered, or even their breathing had been shallower, resulting from the effects of their general health situation. So part of their recovery plan was targeted at general overall strength and health. As such, a pleasant serendipity would take place, and they would look terrific.

The gentleman with history of melanoma told me, that on the day he played football with his 12 year old son, when he removed his shirt his very impressed son said "Whoa! Dad! You're ripped!" Interpreted that meant he looked great.

I had one lady who was 42, tell me she had never looked as good as she did, recovering from a car accident! Her actual words were "I didn't look this good when I was fifteen!"

I won't go into detail about how this affected the rest of their lives, but I'm sure I don't need to tell you this had a dramatic alteration on their self-esteem, an essential personal shift.

When you are given a terminal health diagnosis, as I myself have had, a period of grief for the life you had, closely follows. Whether it is "You have two weeks to live", or "You'll never walk again", you are forced to accept what feels like an unacceptable permanent change, and that alters everything within you; your perspective of yourself, and the life you have is dramatically changed. Your families, your friends, all the decisions you have made that have got you to that place, all this changes in view of this new perspective. And though it seems like the end, bizarrely, it's a great starting point.

Things are not always what they seem.

It is no coincidence that just prior to a person finding their essential gift, or realizing their goals, or achieving their very best, it is often the case that they have recently undergone a major, personal, traumatic event in their life. Some of us need that slap in the face, in order to see more clearly, I guess. Take me for example. That altered perspective changes everything. Some of us need that huge an amount of pressure behind us, to get us over the line.

Take the simple element of carbon. Put under enough pressure, it becomes a diamond.

And so, here I am, telling you, physical healing *is* within your grasp.

And the physical healing is often the least of it.

The human body is astonishing in its power to heal itself. Put in the right environment, the possibilities are beyond our understanding at what the body can do to repair itself. Beyond our understanding, however, does not mean it isn't occurring.

My own clients have and continue to experience healings that appear incredible, sometimes impossible. I have seen an eighty-six year old woman grow more than two inches as her scoliosis affected spine straightened out in a single session. I've seen a disabled child speak, and say "Mum" for the very first time. A stroke victim once again is able to move his arm. A man with a broken foot walks out unaided by crutches. People walk in with cancerous tumours, and leave without them. A woman suffering from drug-induced depression is able to smile, and function again, never again knowing the panic attacks that had hospitalized her on a weekly basis.

This isn't an occasional occurrence either; it is happening every day. Can you even imagine what it's like to wake up each morning, knowing that you will be present for such a moment? For such a healing! I tell you, you are going to love this.

There is medical evidence of these individuals' ailments prior to walking into the room.

And, there is medical evidence of the incredible changes that occurred for these individuals after they had walked out of the room.

What I cannot offer you, is the medical, or even much scientific evidence of what occurred for each of these people whilst in the session itself. Rest assured there is research underway, and as soon as we know, we'll let you know!

Regardless, the healings occur.

What each client experiences however, during their sessions, for this I have thousands and thousands of pages of documentation, as each experience has been as unique as the individual themselves. And those same individuals were keen for you to hear about it. Throughout this book, you will be witness to many client sessions, as I was, so that you may do what I did: learn. Some of the names of the clients are changed, but, by request, most aren't. To each of those clients, so generous in sharing their experiences, I say thank you.

So welcome to a new perspective on healing. My gift to you is to allow you this alternate perspective, by delving into my own experience. After all, this book is really about you… and this extraordinary and truly beautiful gift is available to us all.

I can't wait to see what you do with it!

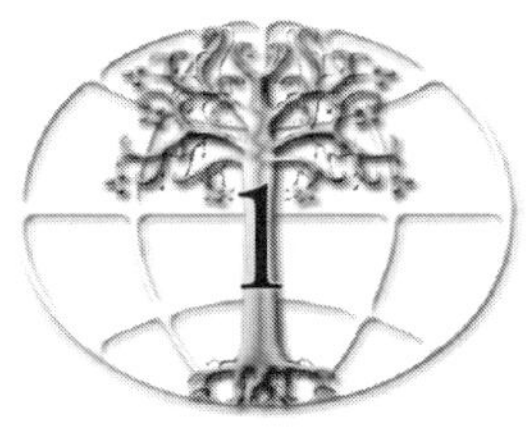

"If you're going through Hell, keep going."
Winston Churchill

The World doesn't revolve around you, you know!

I don't remember a lot of the details about my grandfather. I don't recall a lot of the incidental day-to-day stuff. But I do clearly remember, knowing him so very well, as I have felt it all my life. I was his eleventh grandchild and six years old when he died.

It wasn't long before his death that I was sitting on his lap, amid the colourful multidirectional banter of an extended family gathering. I was leaning back onto his chest chatting to him just so he would answer me and I could feel that great rumble of a voice rolling out of that great mountain of a man. My absolute love and admiration for Popa was full and intense, and even at the age of six I would consciously allow it to envelope me in its ecstasy.

Nearly all of my relatives were somewhat dumbfounded

by me, and as such I was the proverbial "black sheep" and always a "naughty little girl". But I was a pretty little girl with blonde curls and blue eyes, and so they loved showing me off. Provided I didn't speak, or do anything "weird". I was always kept under close restraint, particularly in public; but not by my Popa, he just loved me.

At a gathering only a few years ago, many years after the event, my older cousin recounted to me the conversation I had with Popa that afternoon, upon his lap. He recalled the tears running down Popa's cheeks when I answered.

Popa rumbled, "Lissy, what do you want to be when you grow up?"

And I said, "Wise."

I remember saying it. I remember Pop's silence and, for it made me turn to look at him and bask in his gentle smile. My cousin tells me it was a rare day when he wasn't astonished by me, but on this day I actually silenced the entire family. I can still see the dismayed heads shaking.

Weeks later, I was at school, playing in the playground at recess, when for no reason I knew at all, I burst into tears. When the teacher came over and said, "What is it, Melissa?" I replied, "My Popa just died." She stared at me hard for a moment, then rolled her exasperated eyes and walked away.

I sat down on a bench, desolate and alone beneath the stark branches of a winter tree. My friends were playing around me, but knew not to come to me. I remember feeling like, somehow; I had made the wrong choice.

When my parents picked me up from school that afternoon, they told me that Popa had died; indeed at 10.47am, while I was at recess. I said, "I know." Of course, I was punished for being unfeeling and ill-mannered.

My childhood was not easy. And I was not an easy child.

I'm certainly not proud of that fact, but I do forgive myself now that I am a little wiser.

The truth is I didn't really want to talk about me in his

book. It was a friend working in healing, Paul Ribet that convinced me. He said, "Melissa, who better to help someone that ails, than someone who has been to Hell and back, and then gone back a few times just to see if the climate has changed?"

As a child the confusion was very real. I just could not comprehend the need to conform. Actually I still don't. Norman Vincent Peale seems to understand and put it concisely, *"Conformity is one of the most fundamental dishonesties of all. When we reject our specialness, when we water down our God-given uniqueness and individuality, we begin to lose our freedom. The conformist is in no way a free man. He has to follow the herd."*

Almost thirty years into this life, I finally came to recognize that I don't think like other people, and they don't think like me. My expectations of myself have not really softened at all, but in this discovery, I am far more generous in my expectations of others.

I am an Indigo child. When I read *The Indigo Child* by Jan Tober and Lee Carroll I experienced two things; recognition, and relief. Not only did someone understand that I didn't think like other people think, and didn't seem to have the same social filters; the specialists referenced in the book actually saw merit to this. If you understand or have read about Indigos then you'll be able to laugh at, and comprehend somewhat, the audacious existence that has been, and is, my life.

Of course, it would have been a lot easier if as a child we recognised Indigo children and their differing natures. But my mother was blind in the wilderness to this strangely independent, very strong and apparently defiant child. She was told "discipline her", and when that didn't work, "discipline her harder".

I appeared awkward, I was *painfully* shy, and the majority of my family just couldn't fathom how to communicate with me. And I just couldn't fathom how to get through to them either! I threw tantrums that to this day, only my own children can compete with (sadly for them, as they are dealing with the master). I was grotesquely intolerant of idiots, but rather than let them know it, I simply went within myself. Just didn't answer. I see my son do the same thing now. My son has a physical disability and people, not knowing, assume it must be something to do with his disability. Having been there myself, I see him just choose not to bother himself with such small questions. He too, just goes within.

Not unhappily intrinsic, either. It was, and still is, blissful to escape within and concentrate on the incredible influx of information that I had gathered throughout the day. To filter it, refine, comprehend a little further, or abandon, various interactive information feeds that had occurred. A whole separate adventure lives within our own mind.

I used to, and actually still do, love watching people. I often recall looking at a group of people that I was amongst, from a distance. I could make myself be outside that group when physically I was amid them. And I would watch. And learn.

It wasn't an easy childhood, and a bevy of forces were at work at any moment to assure that status. Bad things happened Bad things. Any single one of these things could have created a victim of me. And with my apparent social ineptitude, I was ill equipped to handle them. Remaining intrinsic, for me, was a defensive action, in the face of the mind chattering chaos of absorbing all the peripherals, as well as dealing with the obvious.

This absorbed, non-communicative existence prompted me to hear the phrase, *"The world doesn't revolve around you, you know!"* more times than I care to remember. Every child hears this phrase at some time. I had it hammered in. It actually wasn't self absorption. To remain intrinsic was a defensive action, in the face of the mind-chattering chaos of absorbing all the peripherals as well as the obvious.

The downfall of my silent defensive strategy came to a head when I started school. Apparently I hadn't been communicating a lot. Despite the fact that an extraordinary amount of activity was always going on within me, I hadn't actually shared a lot of it. As such, when I was at the appropriate age to start school, my mother had placed me in a "remedial" prep class, as they had come to the conclusion that I had some sort of learning disability. I was only in the Prep class for two days when the school put me into Grade Two.

I had been reading since I was three, only Mum hadn't noticed. I certainly hadn't told anyone. I have an extraordinary memory; a true gift that means learning comes very easily to me. (When we meet this is worth remembering, for my memory is long.)

The self discipline to sit down and study was another issue. You would have hated me at school, not studying, getting good grades. But I was so bored and frustrated. I despised being there. Unless I knew I would enjoy the task, I simply refused to complete any assigned homework, and in this my marks did suffer. Homework seemed a pointless exercise of little benefit to any party involved, other than to tax one's time.

I did everything extra curricula during school that I could to stem the boredom and quash the frustration I had at such an inefficient and ineffective system. As such I play a number of musical instruments, speak various languages, etc. The number of rehearsals I attended jazz ensemble, orchestra, senior band, various types of dance, not to mention sports rivalled the entire number of scheduled school classes I had. And I was 11 years old when I developed a plan that would make general education less generic and more effective for the individual. I couldn't understand why the school faculty wouldn't listen; although I do recall the principle saying 'There's something wrong with that girl', as I was leaving his office.

(I'd recommend reading *The Indigo Child* by Lee Carroll

and Jan Tober. This weird existence will make a lot more sense, and you'll know me a lot better.)

Yep, I was the "trouble maker". Not intentionally, but I was certainly perceived as such by the strict faculty at the Catholic school I attended. "Triple F", Father Fred Franklin, the principal of the school, belonged to an order of brothers that had only run all-boy schools. This was their first co-ed school, and he was simply bewildered by me. In a Year Eight report card, my maths teacher wrote, "Melissa has incredible potential. The rest of the class might have too, if she would stop talking to them all throughout the lessons!"

Ultimately I became the school captain. Poor old Father Fred was stuck with me for a whole year. Clearly everyone enjoyed watching this poor man's tortured struggle!

My final year in high school was a nightmare. Most people did five Higher School Certificate subjects in their final year. Because I could, and they were trying to keep me busy, I did four the previous year, and another six in my final year. Ten Math/ Science subjects because, according to my teachers, that would "take me further".

School started in February, and, one week in, I was diagnosed with glandular fever. A month later, I was raped by a young man who apparently had been stalking me for some time (you learn that in hindsight, of course). In April I was diagnosed with Ross River virus which is quite similar to glandular fever, except it also feels like you have hot sand in all of your joints. I wasn't well. I was sleeping 14 – 16 hours a day just trying to stay alive. And school took up all the rest of my time, and what a waste of time it felt like.

Aside from the emotional hurt, I had sustained some significant physical injuries from the rape. This guy had planned the whole thing for months, so he was pretty organised in its execution and ultimately tried to kill me with a piece of wood through the end of which he'd hammered nails.

In Australia, if you suffer trauma or serious illness during your final year at school, they can give you 'special consideration', which gives you some official room for excuse if your marks aren't too hot. A guidance teacher recommended I apply for it. I was rejected because the rape "didn't occur during an examination period". And as for the illness, well, I might get over it before the end of the year.

Regardless, I graduated, and got a university scholarship into Engineering. Great course, just not for me. I was so sick of memorising formulae. For the first time, I seriously addressed career. I had never actually given any thought to what I wanted to do with my life. When I had had that all important appointment with a guidance teacher, and she asked me what I wanted to do when I left school, I answered, "Nothing." These days I'm inclined to think that it was the correct answer. Nothing can be very pleasant, provided money is not an issue.

But I was cruising. I was following the script, the expectations of others. Damn it, I was conforming! Conforming because it was easier than identifying where I needed to go. I left engineering and after a stack of research, decided I wanted to do a Business degree in Marketing. Despite my high marks, they wouldn't let me into the course because all of my subjects had been math/science. (That would be about right, wouldn't it? "*Take me further*", my butt.)

I decided to revert to that Latin proverb: *"If there is no wind, row."*

So I landed in the waiting room of the Dean's office in the Marketing Department, prepared to argue my case. He was too busy, he couldn't see me. So I camped there. I would watch as he walked in and out, calling to me as he passed, although careful not to make eye contact, "No, no, I have an appointment", or "No, I told you my schedule is full!". On the fourth day, he walked out of his office and with a resigned look said, "Melissa, you have five minutes." We both knew the decision, before I'd even entered his office. I started my

Bachelor of Business-Marketing the very next day.

Later that year I was diagnosed with uterine cancer.

As you do with such diagnosis, I went into a state of shock and despair for a couple of days. Then, when I saw the oncologist and they started talking about my treatment, one thing became evident: I didn't have a clue what was going on. I knew I needed to know more about what was happening.

This time I went to the Dean of Science at the University. It was a lot easier to convince him as a nineteen year old with cancer. He tailored a science course in human anatomy/ physiology for me, no doubt specially tailored to help me comprehend my own physical predicament. And there I was; doing a double degree.

I loved it! Just loved it. All my life I have had an affinity with the human body; I could sketch it, sculpt it, paint it, convince my own to do any number of athletics, gymnastics, dance, you name it. I loved the simplicity in its symmetry, yet its utter complexity in symbiotic function.

All my life I have pushed this body of mine. Being tall and muscular, I have always loved the myriad sensations of movement, of exertion, of total relaxation, stretching muscles, even the muscle soreness of over exertion. So yes, I was and still am athletic.

As a child, and even more so as a teenager, I was alarmingly, or as my mother put it, 'embarrassingly' thin. I ate all the time. No eating disorders, nothing like that; just a phenomenal metabolism and huge energy levels. I have always physically "moved", and it has always been my salvation. Even now I weight train and run between 5 and 7 kilometres several times a week. I joke that it's my stress management, but really it's no joke. I was only 12 or 13 when I came to understand that if I didn't get rid of this excessive, pent up energy, it would get ugly. Or rather, I get ugly. So I use it. And with each foot fall, I pound the stress into the pavement.

When I was diagnosed with cancer, for the first time, I

started to train specifically. In all the sports and dance I had done, I had never trained 'sport specific' because I was never just involved in one sport. With cancer I entered the singular sport of survival. I would be at the gym, listening to people's petty bitching about how someone else looked, or acted. A lot of these people were in dire need of an altered perspective! I recall one lady saying, when her trainer asked her what she wanted to look like, "I want to look like her." and pointed at me. I thought, oh no you don't!

Even at my sickest moments with cancer, when the pain and the utter exhaustion were unbearable, I had it in my head that if I moved, I would survive. As long as this body was still in motion, I would survive.

Everyday I made sure I did something physical. There were days when all I could endure was to go from my apartment to my mailbox and back. Each step was agonising, firing hot shots of nausea up my throat. Rushes of fever would leave me lathered in sweat. I would finally fall back in the front door of my apartment, wallow in self pity for a few minutes, then get on with life because I still could. I was still moving.

Under the direction of my doctor, a brilliant guy who had been a bit of a Dougie Hauser, I underwent the usual medical treatments associated with cancer. He had flown through school in record time and started university at fifteen or so. When I met Greg, as my doctor prior to cancer, we had become friends. Instinctually this felt wrong, and no doubt professionally it was, but I loved his company. He was enormously charming, although it was clear to me that I wasn't quite getting the full picture. It didn't worry me at the time. We had the best time together going to major sporting events, dinners and shows at the expense of the drug companies that wanted Greg's business.

In a short space of time, it became clear that the treatments I had been scheduled for weren't working, and the cancer was spreading. When Greg said to me, "We are going to try something new", I never imagined my friend would put me at risk. He put me on an experimental drug, which I was on for two days and then was bedridden for three weeks. Greg got a brand new sports car about a week after I went on this drug. And strangely coincidental was that it never cost me a cent to be on this drug.

After this I had had enough. I put a stop to it all.

I was grey, skeletal, completely bald, not an eyelash to my name, and I felt utterly stripped and devoid. I couldn't eat, although that didn't seem to affect my ability to vomit. My stomach responded to filtered water as though it was curdled milk. The only relief I had at this time was when I closed my eyes; for some reason I felt cooler, safer, calmer. Everything else burned, ached and stung. The chemotherapy left my very veins feeling scraped and charred. You know that feeling you have, when you've spent all night next to a campfire, you can feel that grotty charred sensation in every pore. Well, that was what I felt like on the inside. Bizarrely, I had extraordinary insight to the internal trauma of my own battle raged body.

I was refusing treatment. The oncologist was peeved. He said, "At best, you've got two weeks."

Two weeks to live. Two weeks. I was 20 years old.

So I phoned my parents and told them I had cancer. This probably seems strange, but as I lived alone and some distance from them, I didn't want them to worry. I just wanted to get on with the job of getting over this cancer. Actually, I didn't tell many people about it, because I couldn't tolerate their pity. And I couldn't help them in their distress; I just didn't have the energy. They were *so* angry! But I just didn't have it in me…I had to focus on surviving.

So, I locked myself in my apartment with my cat, Rhubarb. Somewhere on the second day, I just thought, "I don't feel like I'm dying." I wasn't well. I felt like crap, my body was wasted away, just breathing was painful, but I wasn't dying. Perhaps that was why I didn't tell my family or many of my friends; because I knew, within, this would end and I would still be here. So I got up, and got on with life.

I can't explain it. And now I know that it actually doesn't require explanation. The fact that I am still here is enough. My body healed itself.

Within a year I was cancer free.

But the damage was evident. My body was wasted down to its very base elements, and felt foreign to me. I had no strength, restricted movement. Out walking one day I tried to race a friend in a sprint up a hill, and he laughed when he got to the top and I had barely moved from where he left me. He called me "slack", but what he didn't realise is that although I had given it everything I had there was just nothing there. This was a shattering revelation to me. My body had forgotten me! It was not unlike getting into a cab in a foreign country and finding the driver doesn't speak English. We were going nowhere until I could communicate with this body again.

So the very first body I rehabilitated was my own. Sculpted and rebuilt from the wastelands of terminal disease. It felt agonisingly slow, but, in reality, in a matter of months, I had discovered a body purpose-built for *living*.

I was still studying at University, and paying my way by teaching aerobics classes. Sixteen to eighteen classes a week! My body was strong, muscular, capable, and I loved the way it felt again! I was ready for a new challenge.

So I applied to enter the Army. Of course, what else does a young girl do? I wanted to go in at general entry level, as I admired the character at that level, but instead they put me in for Officer Training. Almost a year of psych' tests, medicals (I'll get back to that), exams, hearing tests, the lot. Out of 1200 applicants, 60 got in, and only 3 were women. I was one of the three.

I left you hanging about my doctor, Greg, "doing me

harm". It turned out that Greg had some pretty serious issues, I'm afraid. It turned out that, allegedly, Greg had been having sex with his patients, in his rooms and charging the time to Medicare. What was worse was he was HIV positive, as now are many of the men he'd had sex with. He had, while I'd known him gotten married and had a daughter, thankfully who are not HIV positive. As you can well imagine, all of this was a shock to his wife. He had also, in his charming way, convinced many of his elderly clients to leave their millions to him. And the list goes on. He has been charged with many crimes, including millions of dollars of Medicare fraud. I had been quite the "beard" for my doctor!

No doubt because he was covering his tracks, my medical records disappeared. That is no mean feat, I tell you, and it wasn't just mine alone. Many of his patients have had to deal with this. These records were removed from a number of databases. It's never been a convenient thing, I might add. The only medical records I have left are of a tonsillectomy I had when I was eighteen. However, this worked well for me when I was entering the military.

I was in the Army now.

My mother was horrified, the relatives disbelieving, my father however, having been in the Army himself, said "It will be the making of you." He was so right! It was some of the best times and some of the worst times I can recall.

I had no expectations, except that it would be hard. Perhaps that's why I enjoyed it so much; every day I was pushed to my limit and then beyond it. So every day I had a hugely empowering sense of accomplishment. Even today I still live very much by the Infantry corps motto of *"Improvise, Adapt and Overcome"*.

I later found out that there was a huge betting pool, during my basic training, on how long I would stay in. The longest bet was three weeks. Probably because of my physical appearance, people have a habit of grossly underestimating me.

It wasn't long before my fellow "recruits" figured that out. The guys later confessed that I pushed them all, because I would whip them on the obstacle course, on the firing range, and tactically. We would run at a 10 foot wall and I would make it over first time, one handed, rifle slung. You can imagine the male ego response to that.

And it was that male ego thing that created some of my worst moments in the Army.

Early on it was discovered that I had a talent with weapons. I have a dead eye when shooting, and a love for the mechanism of the weapons we would use. My first love was rifles and individual automatic weapons. No need to worry, it's not some demented crazed obsession. The military ensure that not only are you proficient in handling the weapon, but that you revere it with the utmost respect.

As time came for me to choose a corps, I wanted to go into Armoured; tanks, etc. I mean, why carry the weapon when the weapon can carry you? That and I loved the sound of the 30 cal and 50 cal guns; Beautiful. But justifiably, women aren't allowed in Armoured. We aren't allowed in Infantry either, but that is the corps I entered.

I think Dad was right, I saw so many great guys, grow into great men, in the military. And I'm sure it was the "making of me" too. I made some awesome friendships whilst in the military that last to this day, and could tell you a thousand hysterically funny 'war stories' about our training and exercises, that to this day have tears of laughter rolling down my cheeks.

It was a truly amazing time. But I had to leave…

Something strange had started happening with my balance. One moment I was standing up straight, and then, without any sensation of overbalance at all, I would be lying on the ground. I had headaches, nose bleeds, and a strange taste in my mouth. They thought it was extreme fatigue and sent me to the Regimental Medical Officer. He did tests, blood counts, CT and MRI.

Brain Tumour

They gave me the option of a medical discharge, or I could take leave and 'deal with it'. I chose the latter. But the news wasn't good. It was inoperable. This time I was given 12 months to live.

The death sentence, again.

So many people must simply give up when they hear that. You trust your doctor, you believe what he says to you, so where does that leave your mindset?

When I went back for a check-up three months later, they changed their mind. 'You've probably only got 6 months.

I joked, "What if I'm on a schedule here? You just stripped me of three months!" But I was the only one laughing. "I'm sorry." they said.

I wasn't sorry; I was angry. And as I'm an Indigo, I was *really* angry. I had started to black out, and when I came to the pain was absolutely horrendous. I would crawl very, very slowly, with my head hanging low between my arms to a place where I could rest comfortably, then sleep and sleep.

I was rapidly entering depression and had started to think self pitying thoughts, like, *"Is everyone else's life this bloody hard?"* I went home to my family for Christmas that year, and I could barely crack a smile. Then an amazing gift was put before me...

A friend that I went to primary school with rumbled down our driveway on his Harley Davidson one day. I hadn't seen him for eleven years. He'd heard I was in town and thought he'd drop in. We spent the next couple of weeks purring our way around the beautiful Gippsland Lakes region of Victoria, on the Harley. It was summer and just exquisite.

One afternoon he said. "Let's go rollerblading. I know this guy that is a great skater, we'll go with him. I'll meet you at 8pm down at Lakes Entrance..."

I said, "What's this guy's name?" He said, "Rat."

And I thought, *"Oh great, sounds like a winner!"*

Andrew, aka Rat, was a fantastic in-line skater or rollerblader if you like. You know the guy that does all the tricks and everything? Jumping up onto the rail and back flipping off of it? That's him. At 8pm I drove in the driveway, stepped out of the car, and was met with an appearance that did not match the name.

Andrew skated up and introduced himself. He had hair down to his backside (off his head, not on his body), and wore nothing but a very tight pair of denim shorts. The name "Rat" suited him, until he spoke. He was remarkably articulate, obviously intelligent, warm and very, very funny.

I was not interested in any sort of romance. I was absolutely not looking. After all I had no future. So of course, that is when I met Andrew.

I knew him only two days, and I can remember the very moment when I knew I was going to marry him. I was crossing a street, and was halfway across when it hit me. I nearly got run over in my shock!

My health started getting better. As it turns out, as can happen with illness, it was a great time for me to slow down and re-evaluate things. From the outset, for as long as I could remember, I had been in a hurry. I had to achieve this, try that, beat that system, go there, and in all things, I had to excel. I expected no less of myself. But I had been so busy achieving, that I had not actually been enjoying my achievements. And still, I hadn't discovered where I really wanted to go.

Throughout it all, I was driven. I knew there was purpose. But as yet, not what it was.

Somehow, against all odds, I had started to recover, although it didn't feel like it. Andrew witnessed me blacking out and vomiting. I would be on the floor when I regained consciousness, and Andrew would be lying next to me, his face inches from mine, wet with tears, his brow furrowed with such concern.

Andrew has a wickedly fast sense of humour, and an incredible ability to speak to anyone and make them feel like he was an old friend. Extraordinarily articulate, his humour is intelligent, yet comfortable. At a time when I could barely crack a smile, he had me laughing non-stop.

We had only known each other for eleven months when we got married. No one said to me, "Are you sure? You don't think it's all a bit fast?" Years later when I asked my father about it, he said, "When I saw the two of you together, there was no doubt it was meant to be."

When I look back I should have added a disclaimer for Andrew on the marriage certificate. Andrew entered an existence that was, well in a word, big; my life, never dull and often exhausting. Kryon, in *The End Times,* refers to certain karmic groups, rated according to nature of karmic activity. He numbered these groups from high to low 1-3, 4-7 and 8-10. I was clearly in group 1-3, with a massive amount of fairly brutal lesson thrown at me constantly, in linear time, always overlapping, causing me to appear to others as the perpetual victim. Life just kept happening around me, and friends would say, "How can so much happen in one person's life?"

I am not, now and have never been a victim. Not in my mind. Not in my heart. That is probably the sole reason I still survive.

Eleanor Roosevelt said *"No one can make you feel inferior without your consent."*

Only a couple of months after the stalker got away with raping me and while I was still at school, he raped another girl. After he had attacked me, I could not bear to be touched by anyone, for days. Desperately trying to rid myself of the filth I felt upon me, I had scrubbed, bleached and scorched all physical evidence away. (*Give me a break! I was only 17!*).

When I found out that he had done it again, I went to the girl he had assaulted, and encouraged her to lay charges against him. She said to me, in a wash of tears,

"He's destroyed me; just destroyed me!" I looked at her. "Did he touch your heart?" She shook her head, no. "Did he touch your spirit?" Again she shook her head. "Then he has no hope of destroying you. He can't touch you."

Early on in my life, amid the constant battle between the Indigo that would not conform, and the people that could only cope if I did conform, I learnt that people could only hurt me *if I let them.*

Andrew and I had been married ten months, and had just moved back from the Whitsunday Islands in Northern Queensland, to Melbourne, when I received a phonecall from one of the major hospitals. Andrew, whilst at work with an engineering company, had been crushed by the elevator while working inside an elevator shaft. His injuries were incredible, as you can imagine, and he was fighting for life, and as it turned out, limb.

Multiple surgeries and years of rehabilitation were to ensue. But in true Andrew fashion, he has recovered incredibly, and can now walk. Skating is a thing of the past, but he's compromised by turning his passion to Rally driving (much safer!).

And through this event Life lurched forward, shifting again. It was another big turning point, where the battle became extrinsic for me. There is a great period in your life when you are unencumbered by the responsibility of anyone other than yourself. It is a brilliant, unshackled adventure in time. But now I had to go to bat for my family (consisting of Andrew at the time), and the extrinsic lessons began. The fight was and is no less passionate, but at least now it wasn't always alone.

Writing about one's life is hard! I was told "People need to know who you are, Mel!" Looking back upon what I have shared with you, I see that it is but a fragment of a huge and complex life. As I go on through this journey I have chosen to fulfil, the drama is no less intense, but the journey is one of purpose, and the "powerful play" goes on. If what I have shared appears obnoxious, or negative, or self pitying, my deepest apology for that was not my intent. I assure you writing about myself is the hardest and most uncomfortable part of this book.

Yet it is written for You, with purpose. So much, what I had hoped you would recognise through reading this is that I recognize and know your heart, through my own experiences.

That I can empathise with all of the crap that you have gone through to get to this point; and I respect you for it, fellow warrior, and potential healer that you are.

If you are, right now, in a place of desperation or loneliness, then I invite you to take to heart the immortal words of Sir Winston Churchill, (which I found on my friend Helen's refrigerator on a magnet. Wisdom comes from the strangest places!)

"If you are going through Hell, keep going."

You *are* making the right decisions.

Right now you are exactly where you need to be.

You *are* in the right place. It only gets better from here.

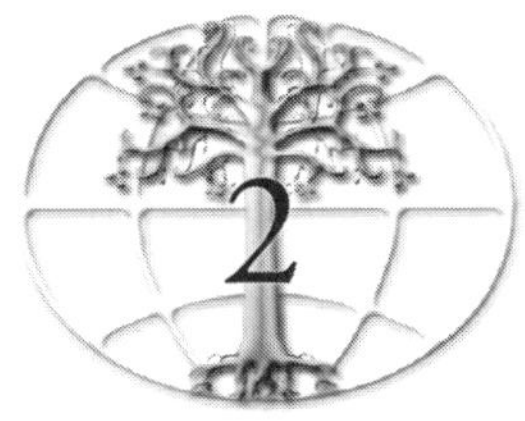

"Your vision will become clear only when you look into your heart. Who looks outside, dreams. Who looks inside, awakens."
Carl Jung

The Initiation

"It's a beautiful little boy!"

My history with cancer dictated a certain infertility which was being utterly contradicted by the beautiful baby they were placing on my abdomen. My exquisitely wonderful, healthy little boy Johnathon Andrew.

Jack.

He didn't cry. He just looked straight into my heart with those deep pool eyes, peacefully, contentedly, but somehow determinedly. It was as if he knew, as he does now, because he still knows.

You go through a pregnancy feeling that baby moving, relishing each kick, shuffle and roll, from deep within your body, knowing that child. Yet that moment when they actually arrive...The moment they take their first breath on this planet and you meet them for the first time, is truly, truly awesome.

Jack went straight to the breast and had just finished feeding when there was a knock at the delivery room door. My father had come to the hospital to see if I was alright, not realizing that Jack had in fact arrived. Something magic occurred when these two met. Jack was twenty minutes old, and his Pop, a tall mountain of a man, was cradling his little namesake with the gentleness only real love knows. Those old eyes looking up staring into the misty eyes of an overwhelmed grandfather, a bond, unspoken and pure, was formed. A certain line was expanding; a certain contract coming into play.

There were congratulations all around as they wheeled us back to the ward. And as everyone does, we showed off our small precious boy as if no-one had ever had a baby before. We were embarrassingly blissful. The next few hours were filled with wonderful friends and family, arriving to celebrate. In flooded an abundance of balloons, flowers and gifts. You could feel the relief of those closest to me, for this body of mine was tired. Illness, which had evolved into disease, had left my body battle weary, and it had struggled under the weight of creation. Toward the end I had started to waste away, losing weight as the baby had flourished and seemed to just eat me alive. I loved being pregnant but it was clear my body didn't and the concern of those nearest to me was evident. This day relief came in the shape of a divine baby, an enormous individual.

Finally there was a lull in the visiting traffic where I was able to simply cherish my boy. He was fussing so I fed him, and went to change his nappy when I noticed his breathing...

His diaphragm seemed to be going into spasm. His breathing was a little wet. Was this normal newborn behaviour? His breathing was normal after delivery. I turned to my husband and asked him to drag out the baby books. No answers there. So I buzzed the nurse, and asked to see a paediatrician.

The midwife gave me that annoying, patronizing look, "You're just nervous, Melissa. You're a new mum, and it's normal that you doubt yourself..."

I broke in "I'm not the panicking kind. We need to see a paediatrician, now. I insist!" These last words I had delivered about three inches from the midwife's face. I had noticed my son's nostrils flaring a little.

"You need to get back into bed and rest, Melissa."

"Please, please get a paediatrician. Please"

"Please get back into bed! I know you're nervous..."

"I am not f...g nervous!" I picked Jack up, and started walking as best I could after twenty-four hours of labour and stitches to boot. "Where do I find a paediatrician?"

Because of my medical history we had chosen a Level 3 hospital, ready for all eventualities. We assumed if anyone might need that level of care it would be me. They brought the registrar down from the Neonatal Intensive Care Unit, because that was who was available at the time. She took a brief look at Jack, picked him up and said to my husband, "You better follow me!" I had enough time to beg Andrew to not leave Jack's side, and they took off at a run!

I was left sitting in the hospital room, alone. No explanation, but a generous amount of fear had been left with me so I wouldn't be lonely. The silence in the room closed in around me. No one came to me to explain, comfort or otherwise. Looking through the doorway of my room, I could see the concern the faces of the midwives and hear the hushed whispers as they glanced with trepidation toward my room.

I tried to get up and follow Jack, shuffling determinedly out of my room and down the hall. But the many hours of labour had taken their toll and I collapsed in the hallway, clinging to the rail on the wall. My heart was shredding within me, the sobs tearing within my chest, the tears falling unaccounted down my cheeks. Nobody was telling me anything!

That was my son! I had been holding that little boy for nine months, what made them think I would let go now? Something was very wrong and I needed to get to my little boy.

Someone saw the grief stricken heap in the corridor (me), and I heard yelling. I was ready to fight to the death to get to my son! I would not be going back to that room! It must have been written all over my face, because the nurses raced to me with a wheelchair, threw me in, and ran, pushing me, all the way to NICU.

Jack had been exposed to bacteria within the hospital, and his newborn immune system had no hope of defence. Seven babies in total that day had been exposed to this bacterium. He had double pneumonia. They had raced him to NICU and started treatment immediately. When he was only eleven hours old, they did a lumbar puncture which confirmed he also had bacterial meningitis. He was fighting for his life.

He was supine in what looked like an open tray, angled upward. Tubes running in and out of this tiny newborn body, taped across his face, aggravating his soft, petal-like skin. Each breath was a struggle, only the energy to survive. It was one o'clock in the morning when they assured me that he was stable, and wheeled me back to my room to rest.

Four o'clock in the morning the nurses exploded into my room.

"The baby has taken a turn for the worse! We have to get you to NICU!" How much worse could it get?

He was sixteen hours old. Jack had gone into a massive seizure, his entire system trying to shut down. They couldn't get any lines in, and the panic on the faces of that extraordinary medical team was evident as they parted so that I could be next to my son. They told me I needed to speak to him; he needed to hear my voice.

I looked down at his grey stiff, little body. No detectable

heartbeat. Not breathing. I touched his sweet, soft cheek, and said "Hi Angel." And his little head turned toward me.

I started to talk to him. It was our first serious conversation, and believe me there was no brave hero or courageous mother in me, when I said to him that if this was too much, he could leave. I won't even try to describe the utter desolation and despair in my heart at the thought of losing my child. Only experience lends you that kind of pain. My heart only knew utter desolation at the thought of him dying; the pain is still real for me now. But the battle ahead of him was brutal. Please, don't mistake it. I was not spiritually evolved, I was not an outstanding woman by any means, there was truly nothing heroic about it.

I loved my son. I had from the moment the incredulous doctor said "You're pregnant!" I didn't understand why he would leave so soon, why he needed to go now. How could any mother's heart understand? But I knew something big was at play here, and the decision was Jack's.

They worked frantically as I sang and spoke to him. Finally, I heard the magic words, "He's stable." A nurse touched me on the shoulder tenderly "Would you like to call your husband?" I looked at the clock. It had been two and a half hours.

Not even a day old.

Seven babies had been exposed to these bacteria. Jack was the only one to survive.

Exactly three years later, on Jack's third birthday, I met one of those significant friends that come in and out of your life with a single purpose: to direct you.

I was reading an article about some fairly extraordinary work a gentleman had been doing with healing in America. This article was vague but about the possible effect of quantum frequencies on human cellular regeneration. I read this and something within me clicked over, not unlike the arrow on a compass. I burst into tears, not really understanding why

I was so overwhelmed, I turned to Andrew and said "We have to find this man." Bursting into tears is not common practice for me, the importance was evident, so Andrew read the article and said "Whatever it takes. We'll find him." We had no money to spare, and it looked like we needed to go the United States, but we both knew this was incredibly important. We started placing phone calls around the world trying to find him, only to discover that three days later he would be lecturing in Melbourne, the city where we lived.

So I went. The lecture was being held at a facility I wasn't familiar with, so when I arrived, I was at the wrong entrance for the facility and walked in at stage level. Immediately there was a small smattering of applause, as a few in the audience assumed I was the presenter. I took rapid evasive action and dove for a seat in the front row.

The crowd surprised me, to say the least. I had a double degree in science and had worked in the rehabilitation and sports industries. I expected other such professionals to be there. Honestly, part of my anticipation of these things is the incredible education that sprouts from the incidental acquaintances you meet. So I was expecting doctors, specialists, physiotherapists, etc. However, the incidental education I was to receive was not at all what I had expected. Instead, the audience was filled with an extraordinary mix of peoples, having all manner of injury and illness, all of them wanting to be healed.

The lady next to me had very bad chronic fatigue syndrome, and I spent most of the time asking her if she was alright. She was all bundled up and yet still shivering, and if I needed to know where this bloke was, all I had to do was watch her watering eyes as they tracked him. She needed help, she wanted to be healed, and this man was the "miracle healer" she had been waiting for. (*Miracle healer? Am I in the right place?*) I listened to her impassioned yearning throughout the presentation. All I heard of the lecture was at the end, when one of his assistants responded to an audience question "…No, I'm afraid he doesn't do private sessions. However, he will be teaching a workshop in two weeks time here in Melbourne…"

And I thought, 'Bloody charlatans! Here they go trying to rip us off with their bloody new age workshops!' That would be right! What an incredible waste of all of our time. This was Jack's third birthday and his mother is in here, listening to this!

Andrew was just outside with Jack, 3 (just that day), and our eldest daughter Colby, 9 months. I could hear Andrew happily chatting to someone, so I turned to the lady next to me to see if she needed assistance to leave. She was devastated. She had been hoping this man would work on her. As we talked and I consoled, the beautiful woman Andrew had been talking to, introducing herself as Savannah, walked over to me and interrupted, "Can you hang around for a while, sweetie? He wants to talk to you." Savannah indicated toward the gentleman that had just been presenting. I was suspicious

"Why?" I could see this man watching us through the crowd.

Andrew leaned in, smiling and said, "We can hang around, can't we?"

I couldn't believe it! "Why?"

A voice said, "You have a gift for this." I looked up into the eyes of a man who would turn out to be a key friend on this road of discovery. And so we hung around.

I didn't really know why I was there, but I **knew** I had to be there. I assumed at the time that it must have been for Jack. You see the previous three years, since Jack's arrival had been laden with many a battle on my son's behalf.

Jack has a severe level of spastic quadriplegia cerebral palsy. He acquired it from the trauma to his brain from the bacterial meningitis. He's not what you'd call "text book" cerebral palsy, (although what the hell that is I don't know). Jack's a very handsome little boy, with clear speech and all of his spastic tone is reactive tone. This means that you don't really see the CP until he first tries to move, then his body rejects the idea and fights him, and Jack fights back. Man, does he fight back! To do anything; to breathe, to eat, to speak, let alone sitting, walking, etc. I tell you he is one extraordinary person.

He's also intellectually brilliant. He started reading when he was 2 (we're yet to figure out where he learned to), and has a phenomenal memory, particularly for music. From as early as 15 months old, he would hear a piece of music once, Mozart, Ben Harper, Jimi Hendrix, and could sing it back note for note. Then in sheer contradiction, the last two years have seen our son develop an incredible battle with communication. He has great speech, but to get it all in the right order is a battle. He tells us there's "too much noise" in his head. He's quite the adventure as a son.

We've watched in the gifted role of parent, calling this child our son, as he reaches out to everyone he meets and changes them. What I'm talking about here is not about disability. It is a lot of fun watching various reactions to a child in a hot looking fluorescent yellow wheelchair, and in his disability there are lessons for everyone. But that's the least of Jack's work. Jack has a presence and ability to affect people as I've never seen before. People change because they meet Jack. He is all love, and more and more I recognize just how indulgent and patient he is with me, as my teacher.

I'll try to explain a complex situation to him, and he'll look at me quietly, and say "I know, Mum." Not condescendingly, or cheekily, just patiently waiting for me to recognize. Those that can see auras tell me his is huge and white, pink and gold. Those that can see spirits, see an enormous crowd with him. But if you haven't recognized your gift yet, rest assured you would still see Jack as he is, for he is beautiful.

My friend, who "doesn't do private sessions", asked us if

he could work on Jack. Of course, we said yes, (who wouldn't?) and my initiation began.

During the session as he worked on him, Jack was singing a favourite song when he suddenly stopped singing, and pulled the man toward him. He reached up and kissed him on the forehead (right on the third eye) and said, "No thank you, I'm alright." And sure enough, there was no physical change in Jack.

Apparently this "miracle healer" was almost as disappointed as I. Two days later, the phone rang and he was asking if they could work on Jack again. In a calculating move, he had asked Savannah to call me. The bond between Savannah and I had been instant; familiar and warm. From that moment when she had introduced herself, I'd felt like saying "Where have you been? I've missed you." This rather than the usual rudimentary salutation. Larger than life, gifted in spirit, Savannah embodied both gift and guide throughout this crucial turning point.

So when she called again, we went. They filmed this session for a television show. Jack had trouble staying still during the session, and was chatting about "The birdies are everywhere, Mum! Look at the birdies!", so the two of us started singing a song about lying straight and still. I recall hearing a lot of sniffing and when I looked around everyone had tears running down their faces; the cameraman, the sound guy. I turned back to my son in time to see him grab the gentleman's hand as he was working, held it and said;

"It alright, you know. I'm okay." And again there was no change.

Jack was the first to show me, before I'd even begun in this work, that people can and would refuse healing. This was a brutal, heartfelt lesson for me, as it had to be for me to recognize the magnitude of the role I was here to fulfil, and that it was not for me to interfere with any individual's journey if it wasn't appropriate. With Jack it was a decision he was aware of, whereas most people are consciously unaware of the road before them. My journey continued…

I spent the next ten or so days with this team, embracing an introduction to this gift of healing, as they generously imparted as much as they understood of it. I didn't learn a lot about the frequencies from them, but I was most certainly introduced to the concept that these quantum based frequencies were *readily available*, for *all* of us. I learnt how to utilize the ever present buzzing in my hands, how to start working on a body, what to feel, where to look, how to work with it a little.

The day after I met them, my neighbour, Lynn, came over. She had laryngitis, and had completely lost her voice. Andrew told her some version of what had happened and what I was doing, and, courageously, she lay on our dining room table while I worked on her for about five minutes. I really had no idea what I was doing, but I could feel the rush of "energy". I moved my hands slowly about her throat and head, feeling the pockets of "pull" in and kind of around my hands. I would stop and stay at a place where there was a pressure sensation in my hands. Then when I no longer felt that "pull" I would move to another area until I felt that sensation again.

From my side of it, it felt like never-ending silk scarves were being quickly pulled through the palms of my hands, up though my arms, shoulders and neck, and out through the top my head. Two more "scarves" were constantly moving through the soles of my feet, up my back and again out through the top of my head. Even then, I knew this wasn't *of me*. I was not the healer here. Yet strangely for me at the time, I was not afraid of these frequencies.

I looked at Lynn and what was happening to her. Her eyelids were flickering madly, and her breathing was shuddering and short. Beneath her closed eyelids her eyes were slowly oscillating from side to side. Her head moved rapidly from side to side intermittently.

Andrew was watching intently, but with a bemused smile upon his face. You got the feeling he knew something he wasn't telling me, and he was truly enjoying watching it unfold. (What had they been discussing while I was resisting all of this?) To his credit, not once did Andrew ever doubt what I was doing. He never questioned it, or denied me access to the avenues I had to go down. In hindsight, Andrew knew, long before I did, that this was what I had to do. What I was here to do. His belief and support was priceless.

Lynn's head was still moving about, but now her eyes opened, although it was clear that she hadn't meant them to be. Her strange, unfocused gaze was a little unsettling. That was enough for me! I placed my hand on her shoulder. She sat up, and looked at me and said, "My throat doesn't feel any different. I don't think it worked but its okay, Mel. You'll get it!" Before she realized her voice was completely restored! Trust me; I was more shocked than her. But Lynn was so excited.

Lynn, a professional renovator, had some furniture removalists at her house that day. She'd come over for a cuppa (that's Australian for "cup of tea") to escape the chaos. She was paying these guys by the hour, and one had broken his foot the day before. You can see her motivation here, right? She ran out to get him. In short order he hopped in on his crutches while Lynn gave him a rundown that I was a "healer". So I worked on his foot…and in ten minutes he walked out the door, pain free, and actually forgot his crutches. Once Lynn picked her jaw up off the floor, she took them to him.

Not even a day old.

Something was afoot.

That same night I returned to the hotel to have part two of an *axiatonal* procedure completed. One of the sources that attempts to explain this healing process, and in particular this axiatonal procedure, is *The Keys of Enoch; the book of knowledge.* In order to learn of it and its purpose Chapters *3: 1:*

4(the "what") and, *3: 1: 7(the "how")* were quite informative for those following at home.

It was recommended that I have it done. When my friend had had this procedure done to him, in short, he awoke the next day with an unprecedented and inexplicable healing ability. I can certainly relate to that!

This procedure is an **Axial Initiation**™. An enormous personal shift, this procedure enables unique vibratory levels and frequencies for healing and ultimately, for our own personal evolution. Enormously personal, unique for each individual, this procedure enhances your knowledge both of yourself, and at a higher level, of the journey ***you*** are upon.

It's done over two days and the cost was $333. The money alone made me take it seriously. I remember the first stage, for my part, but I have no memory of the second stage or of the four days after it.

During the first session, the "quiet in my mind" was anything but. If there has ever been a time when my head hasn't been moving at warp speed it's unbeknownst to me. So to quiet the mind and "check out" was my greatest challenge during this. For some reason, apparently just after he started the whole thing, as I was trying to "check out" and stop thinking, I had a flash back from an episode of M*A*S*H. For the fans of M*A*S*H, it was this moment where Henry Blake is searching for something in Hawkeye's tent, and he shakes the flu as he's looking up, and gets covered in black soot. What I remember was the effort I went to not to laugh. What was reported later was that I laughed and laughed out loud for ages. Damn.

I was chilled, really chilled, and quite self-conscious because I could feel myself shuddering all over. The sensation then changed to a heavy buzz that felt like it was just under my skin, uniformly, and moving deeper within. This was not a light tingling. I was sure you would be able see my skin rippling with such fierce activity beneath it. Disconcerting? Yes.

It felt like something was taking me over! I started to question what would happen when this noisy buzz actually reach skeleton depth. At this point I was forced to make a decision; I could get up, and say "No thanks. You're all a pack of nutcases." And leave. Or I could trust my own heart and let go.

I chose the latter.

The moment, I mean the *moment* I had made that decision, I saw a huge array of colour rushing past me, as if I was propelled down (dare I say it?) a tunnel of some sort. It wasn't a solid tunnel, but instead, very like the television depiction of a wormhole. Different coloured clouds of light formed the shape of a tunnel around me, and it undulated incredibly up and down and around. This ride was incredibly fast, the colours flying past me, and not so smooth I might add, for when I finally slowed as I arrived at where I needed to, I felt physically nauseous.

I had arrived at a place, or rather at a colour; an indescribable (although of course I will try to describe it) blue. Enveloped and cradled within an iridescent, pearlescent blue that had no structure, yet I knew it was spherical. It had no size, no beginning or end to it.

More than that was the *feeling* of arriving there, the emotion. If you could physically enter the most generous of smiling eyes, that is what it felt like. My tortured heart rested, my busy mind stilled, and I was just… feeling. A blissfully ecstatic, soulful entwining that I never wanted to leave. My journey continued there for some time, and much happened.

Then suddenly I was brought back to a basic physical awareness when someone took hold of my arms. Two hands, one on each arm, had taken hold of my forearms. And I was thinking "What is he doing? Isn't he supposed to be drawing lines off the body?" I was furious, I'm talking tantrum-sized furious, as I had not wanted to leave the "blue". Five minutes later (I think) he was still holding my arms. By now, I was only just stopping myself from sitting up and bawling him out. I mean really, I'd paid $333 for this, and I could have held hands with anyone for free! Sometime later, he touched me on the chest to indicate the session was over.

I opened my eyes, and only then realized that the whole time, when I thought I had been there for I could hear him moving about, hear the storm raging outside, I hadn't in fact been in the room. When I opened my eyes was when I realized something big had happened. A moment later, I recognized that I could still feel the hands holding my forearms, only I was physically alone in the room. And the two hands were different; one was large, strong and somehow masculine, the other finer and smaller. To this day I can still feel them there.

That night I awoke at 3.33am and, without thinking, I got up with purpose, feeling like I had something to do. I wandered into the kid's room (out of habit no doubt), both were sleeping peacefully. What woke me up? I felt edgy, like an unknown equation was upon me (which of course it was) but I talked sense to myself, logically. I silently chastised myself for my own melodramatic response, and went back to bed.

I have no real memory of the second stage. I can't even tell you how I got there, let alone how I left. At this juncture, you might recall that I have a fairly extraordinary memory, so this is no small statement. For the few days after the process was finished, I have no memory. I know I functioned normally, attending to appointments and family as I normally would have, but I simply have no recollection of what and how I did any of it, during those days.

When my brain did kick back in, I was different. More awake, more aware. But more incredibly to me was that for the very first time in my life I had something I had always sought…contentment. A peace had arrived within my heart that I had not known before. A smoothness where before there had been jagged edges.

Later in my experience a client finally gave good description to this feeling. She told me "It's like your heart has a huge "ease"." I love that. It's spot on.

This process of Axial Initiation™ is an enormous and very unique shift for an individual. When I am doing this for someone there are times when, even though I am essential as the tool through which this procedure is applied, it can feel like I am intruding. What each individual goes through is as unique and transcendent as the person themselves and it brings in whatever they need on their journey. It enhances them in every way, truly bringing them "into their own". For me it accelerated the flow of these frequencies, completely altered my perspective and my life, (not to mention the lives of those around me!) and that was just the start of it.

There are never two alike. And it is never small. I am absolutely awestruck by the sheer magnitude of it. My respect for both this procedure, and for the person choosing to take this step, has never waned. Nor has my gratitude for it. It is enormously beautiful, as it was for me. That much I do remember.

The effect of this procedure on me was instantaneous. It had an effect very much like the "drop in the ocean". In our family my husband was the head of the house, and I was the centre of it; neither role subservient to the other. So you can imagine how this affected our family, our household, our business, friends, the grocer, my hairdresser... and the ripples keep going out.

It was a palpable change. We had an amazing gift come to us in the form of a respite carer called Karen. She would come to us for a couple of hours a week to give me a little break although we spent most of the time chatting anyway. Karen had only recently made some fairly radical changes in her own life, and while she at this stage wasn't sure where she was going, she knew these decisions were true to her heart. Unlike me, she trusted that. She is truly wonderful. Eventually I had the privilege of doing both her and her husband's Axial Initiations.

Karen arrived for her shift on the same day I worked on Lynn and her removalist just as the removalist was walking comfortably out the door. Karen looked a little perplexed as she watched him leaving, then came inside, took one look at me and said "Oh my god! What has happened to you?" Apparently I looked entirely different. And being in the room with me felt changed too. I honour the role Karen played in this transition, as it was not dissimilar to the backboard in basketball: just as it seemed all over and I'd convinced myself that for some unknown reason I had become delusional, she'd rebound the reality back into play.

About ten days after I'd met my friend and his team, about a week after my own Axial Initiation™, I attended their 'workshop'. There I learnt a lot about people! This was a crowd I'd never experienced before; a New Age crowd. Reiki masters were many, and every type of alternative "healing" method and procedure was already represented in that room; Thought Field Therapy, Reiki, Bowen, Pranic, Crystal, Kahuna, massage therapists of all types, and more. It caused quite a stir, when we were asked to each introduce ourselves and I stood up and said, "Hi, I'm Melissa Hocking. I'm an Anatomical Physiologist. Until recently, I was an officer in the Australian Army. And most importantly, I am a wife and mother." In a nutshell.

New words entered my vocabulary like *"modality"*, and new experiences abounded. There were some truly amazing, genuinely gifted people in that room, sharing wisdom, and generously sharing themselves. I was learning so much. An unexpected bonus was that I also had numerous unsolicited readings from various psychics and clairvoyants. Someone would walk up to me and say, "Do you know you have nine spirits working with you at the moment? One of them is a child." I replied, "That would be right! I thought I left the kids at home." And we would laugh.

Inside though, I was reeling. I felt like I was clinging to

my sanity by my fingertips. The changes were occurring at warp speed. I wasn't sleeping for the burning and buzzing in my hands, arms and upper body which had started the day I "hung around". I was seeing things that in this life I had been conditioned to fear. People that weren't in the physical, shall we say, would walk toward me and take my hand or sit next to me, and frankly scare the heck out of me. These were not spirits that were "stuck" or "ghosts" if you will, but spirits that apparently just wanted to say "hi". A very confronting battle with fear had started. I had anticipated physical healing, certainly, but this spiritual element…

In that crowd I also experienced an element of hostility that was new to me. The few close friends I made there were defending me as only friends would, as apparently jealousy became an issue. Savannah became my sanctuary. I was an attending novice in this crowd. I thought these people would be spiritually evolved and certainly above such petty rubbish, but it seemed I was wrong. In fact, I would venture to say that in some regards ego was a greater issue in this audience. Everyone there wanted to be special, to be gifted, and to be better than everyone else, and above all, to be recognized as such. Normal human behaviour, just amplified.

On the Sunday morning as I walked up the stairs to the last day of the workshop, much to my own surprise I quickly turned the other way and ran into the Ladies room. I hid in a cubicle in a fog of uncertainty, as I pretty much lost control. I started to shake violently and the tears flowed, my heart was pounding and I did not want to leave that cubicle. Actually looking at the words now, it looks pretty much like a panic attack, doesn't it? It wasn't, but it looks like one. All the time I was thinking, *this is just some new age workshop. What is my problem? Just walk in there and finish it, Melissa!* But I had never felt so alone, just desolate, and strangely, kind of, abandoned.

I was aware that I had crossed a line of sorts, but I couldn't remember making the choice to do so, a difficult concept for a choleric individual. It wasn't about the healing gift, it was about the absolute abandon from a world I knew, and functioned pretty well in, into a world I had always known but couldn't recall the techniques to survive. I was despondent and terrified, and really not sure why. I was trying to remember who I was, or at least *how* I was. These changes were occurring at the very core of me, a deeper level that I had ever known in this life.

The next day my friend and his team left the country and I entered the abyss. I have always and will always appreciate that they did introduce this gift to me, and I am always grateful for it, but beyond this we had discovered between us a true friendship. To have such great friends who had walked similar paths and could empathize to at least some degree was priceless... when they could. I knew what my friend's schedule was like, the demand he was constantly under, and knowing that, I didn't want to bother him. But, of course, occasionally it became too much and I did.

I would call and say, "Something weird is happening." and go into it. I would usually finish with "Is this normal?" How he did not blatantly laugh at that question, I don't know. Regardless his answers were bloody frustrating. If it wasn't "I don't know", (one of my own common answers these days), then it was, "You already know the answer to that Melissa, don't you?" (Apparently not) or, "Keep going, Melissa. You'll be okay."

My wonderful friend, he knew, as I do now, that the truest education would come from within. That's why I had to go over the precipice, into the abyss.

The close up into the life I now lead, the path I now go down, I would not ordinarily share it with you. It is personal and it hasn't been easy. In the past couple of years it has become evident that people need to see the battle that went on within me so that they don't feel alone in their own transition. Wisdom is born of experience, and I would rather you could share in mine than walk the road alone as I did.

That being said, I recognize that I do in fact continue to walk the road alone. A great friend and inspiration to me, Scott Alexander King, reminded me in his book, *Animal Dreaming*, that in my commitment to pass this on to you I had chosen to walk this spiritual path alone. For the only way I can truly assist anyone else, is to take on the lesson myself and be true to the contract I not only agreed to, but orchestrated. I am fortunate that I have great friends and family that walk a similar road beside me, and my gratitude for them never wanes. When you get right down to it however, this contract, this purpose, is my own responsibility.

A year or two into this I was attending a conference in Sedona, Arizona, and I was tormented by the choices I had before me. Honestly, I was about walk away from this work. I'd absolutely had enough of the small minded and unprofessional behaviour of the people I was *trying* to work with. My business manager, Helen (very professional and great friend), was out shopping (while I was working!) when a man, a total stranger walked up to her and said, "I need to meet your friend."

Helen said, "That would be Mel." By this stage Helen was used to the amazing adventure that is my life.

He was Native American, and he offered to take us into the Grand Canyon, to places that the general public wasn't able to access. Helen arranged our schedule to enable us to go with him. It meant missing a crucial day of the conference, and I was expected to attend a dinner that evening, so I couldn't believe she had arranged this. And yet we went.

Asked to meet him at 6.45am in the Hotel foyer, I was at the desk telling the staff that if anyone asked where I was, they should just say they didn't know. Then I heard Helen greeting someone. I turned around and looked at this man for the first time, and I fell back a couple of steps. I didn't know who he was, but I could feel how big he was. He introduced himself as Two Bears.

A man of integrity (a hard thing to find for me at the time), a great sense of humour, my god he made me laugh, but more than that, a great sense of peace. Two Bears had a calm that radiated wisdom. This, amid all his jokes and ironic anecdotes! But in his presence all at once you felt totally humbled, and yet secure in an embrace, a blissful, soulful embrace, warm and comfortable.

We arrived down on the banks of the Colorado River, and had a delicious lunch, before he turned to me and said, "You need to tell me about the work you are doing." Two Bears, as it turned out, was a Sioux/Hopi Holy man. On this day he brought it all home to me, as I so desperately needed it to be. On this bright and brilliant day, I ended up doing a healing session on a Native American (he told me I could call him an Indian) Holy man, on the banks of the Colorado River in the middle of the Grand Canyon, beneath an incredible red rock formation known as the Guardian Maiden. He taught and shared so much, because it was what we were there, together, for. The one day in this life where he would play the role he had determined to play. At the end of the day, as we parted at the hotel with huge hugs and many blessings, he turned to me and said,

"Melissa. Walk *your* path, and walk it true." Then turned and walked away.

And I went to the dinner that night committed, come what may, to the task I am here for.

Allow me to share the wisdom I received, with you.

Above all else walk your path, and walk it true. For it will benefit others even more, as well as benefit you. Seek and live by your own truth as you know it. Know your heart, your truth, and then whatever the situation, you will know, If it doesn't ring true, it isn't.

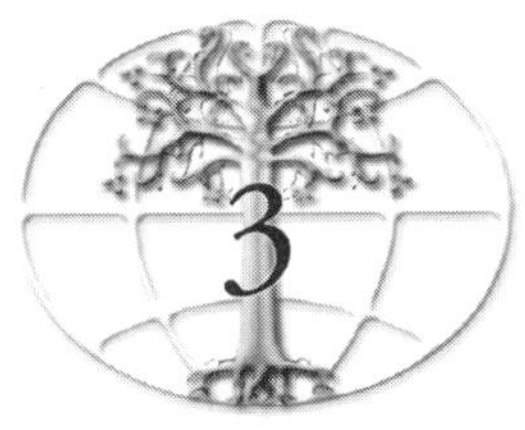

"See yourself and what you will become"
Aristotle

Quantum Frequencies?

This process of healing is a non-intrusive, hands-off form of healing whereby a body is safely immersed within quantum based frequencies and is then able to instigate and facilitate an appropriate healing for itself.

This process of healing is the **Quantum Bioenergetic Balancing Technique**™.

Quantum weirdness? The first time I heard this phrase, from a physicist mind you, I thought he was being humorous (I *know. A scientist?.*) Quantum physics and quantum phenomena are weird, to a huge degree, and it was easy to accept that this physicist was as baffled as the mere laymen so he, too, would call it just plain "weird".

I enjoy classical physics and general relativity. I am one of those people that asks "How?" and enjoy that it can be shown to me quantifiably. When I asked why light refracted in a certain way, or how a uniform acceleration could be achieved, the answer was linear and definite. Throughout my education I embraced physics through mathematics and science. Through formula and pattern and predictable behaviour, the end was determined, and the query completed. I do like symmetry, so you can understand how I liked physics.

Gary Zukav, author of *The Seat of the Soul* says *"We are evolving from a species that pursues external power, into a species that pursues authentic power. We are leaving behind exploration of a physical world as our soul means of evolution. This means of evolution, and the consciousness that results from an awareness that is limited to the five sensory modalities, are no longer adequate to what we must become"*

Modern physics demonstrates that physical matter is simply energy vibrating at different rates. By altering the rate of vibration in the physical, the fundamental elements of physical matter's structure can actually be altered. Einstein once stated, "*We may therefore regard matter as being constituted by the regions of space in which the field is extremely intense...There is no place in this new kind of physics for the field and matter, for the field is the only reality.*"

Quantum mechanics in its definition tells us any end is possible. This suggests the possibility of any number of resulting moments and hence any number of possible futures. Each of these possibilities lies dormant, awaiting the instigation that would allow it to unfold as it follows the immeasurable, yet evidentiary (for the most part) quantum pattern.

Quantum physics relates to the dynamics of atomic and subatomic systems founded in earlier discoveries of quantum theory and wave mechanics. More recently, within the last two decades or so, string theory, a mathematical theory that provides a unified structure to explain the properties and behaviour of elementary particles and fundamental forces at the subatomic level, revolutionised quantum mechanics.

Then a gentleman, Edward Wittel, brought harmony to this theory of the frenetic, immeasurable building block of nature (the string) when he mathematically unified string theory into "M theory". And "M" theory is taking us into new dimensions… quite literally.

While this explanation is brief, the discoveries under the equations of quantum mechanics are truly exciting. From multiple parallel dimensions, or "membranes", to the possible interdimensional leaps of the travelling graviton, any end does seem possible.

Gary Schwartz and Linda Russek in their book titled *The Living Energy Universe*, discuss that all that exists is alive, has memory, and is constantly evolving. As they put it, *"What goes around, evolves around – over and over, changing with every cycle." In this title, regarding quantum effect, they state "If we were looking for a place to find spirits and life, the quantum level would be the place to look."*

What is it?

Quantum BioEnergetics is actually far less complex than it sounds. It is the use of readily accessible **quantum** frequencies, via the human **energy** anatomy, for the purpose (in this balancing technique) of aiding the **biology**.

When a healing session is facilitated in this balancing technique by utilising these quantum frequencies, a healing process is initiated triggering a whole body entrainment. This vibratory entrainment, these frequencies, we believe enable a communication via the human energy anatomy, wholly elevating the cellular vibration and awakening the ability of the human biology to heal itself.

This process of healing offers us an enormous and unprecedented ability to heal ourselves, and, should you choose to do so, to reach out and heal others. This process, through a vibratory whole body entrainment, appears to be assisting the human energy anatomy to shift higher, to vibrate at a higher rate and embrace what was dormant knowledge from within, and to accept unprecedented healings on many levels.

These frequencies are *all encompassing.* Rather than a substance or an entity unto itself, or perhaps more alarming, something superior to everything else, these frequencies are a *process* of ever moving energies. They exist as a constant and evolving continuum of energy. They exist wholly at a quantum level. Why quantum? Linear measurements, even in our rapidly evolving and progressive science, is inadequate to either measure or house these frequencies, for there is no distance, no time frame. Now is all we have, and it is *now* where this exists.

These frequencies are born of Light. J.J. Hurtak, Ph.D., author of *The Keys of Enoch; the book of knowledge,* refers to ***light*** as *"the grid through which and by which all higher forms of energy are transduced so that man may receive them."* Light is an all encompassing information web through which all frequency is constantly communicated. Light is ultimately a construction of information rather than energy as we, the laymen, would understand "light".

In the duality that it is to be human, with our linear perspective of energy, the visual you're probably experiencing in your own mind right now is a beam that has everything in it: all types of energies and interrelated frequencies, systems of communication with a clean cut binary explanation. Right? What makes us uncomfortable is that real light, not the stuff that happens when you flick the switch on, no, I mean that all-encompassing light is more likely a spherical resonant shimmer, boundless, immeasurable and infinite.

The beauty is that you don't need to do anything special or even ritualistic to manifest these frequencies. They continue to flow through us, within each and every particle in existence, in our very cells, in the vibration of the DNA matrix, within us. There is a tangible, verifiable communication housed in the very fundamentals of biology that we suspect is now being accessed through this vibratory process.

There is no denying that these frequencies can also in some part fit the classical definition of energy. As they should, if they are to be all inclusive, all-encompassing. They clearly and evidently do have an electromagnetic presence. And why not? Magnetism relates to all that is synergetic around you; the earth, your own biology, and your DNA are just a few examples. An increased flow of these frequencies is bound to affect any stationary electrically based object that may be exposed to them.

Often when in session, teaching courses, or lecturing, I'll blow a light globe or a fuse in the room. For this reason we usually take a store of light globes with us. I can walk past the amplifier and turn it off while it flashes with "overload". It can be a little inconvenient too, for example my mobile phones (cell phones) usually only have lives of three or four months before they fizzle out.

Other than to explain this process to you as "frequencies", which they are, I have no other name for this transference whatsoever. And I don't need to title them. Yet I do see evidence in the healings before me that occur in session as I assist them. That is why what I teach and facilitate is **Quantum BioEnergetics.**

This process of healing is a non-intrusive, safe form of healing whereby a body is immersed within quantum based frequencies and is then able to instigate and facilitate an appropriate healing for itself.

This immersion is not a "procedure" or "method", it is a *process.* There is no official protocol or preliminary procedure which is why medical professionals, counsellors, practitioners of various modalities are able to easily adapt and utilize this to their clients' and patients' benefit.

The facilitator's body, instrumentally acting as the vehicle through which this light and information, these frequencies are transferred, effectively initiates, then utterly immerses the client body within frequency and the process begins.

That which occurs from this point on is mere speculation and my own perspective. I mentioned earlier that at this stage I have little scientific evidence to offer until we know more of what and how the "gaps" in DNA are being reactivated, more about quantum evolution and evidentiary "measurable" facts, and more about us. I can tell you we have some extraordinary research happening as I write, and the book that will follow this one; "*A Healing Evolution*" should have some exciting discoveries and results to impart.

Regardless, thousands of client sessions, facilitated for an enormous range of injuries and health problems, are evidentiary in the effective application of these extraordinary quantum frequencies.

A fundamental element in this is that it is not that everything that exists **has** fields of vibration but that everything that exists ***is*** fields of vibration. Of course this demands recognition that the human body as an individual vibratory energy system, relates with the wider framework that is the universal energy system.

Why does the biology respond so? In my mind I have little doubt that the communicator, DNA, able to communicate through higher vibrational levels, is connecting with that innate and all knowing memory within; cellular memory.

So many are teaching and talking of cellular memory these days, for it is where we are at in our evolution. Some are showing us this from a scientific and scholarly approach, bringing forth education from history (yes, this does appeal to me). Some, such as the Dalai Lama, bring wisdom to it from heart and spirit. Many approach this extraordinary concept from varying aspects. And then there is my own approach from yet another perspective; **from within you.**

All of us are right. Because each us is enabling you to reach out from wherever you feel most comfortable, in order to reach the wisest, and most demanding, teacher of all; You.

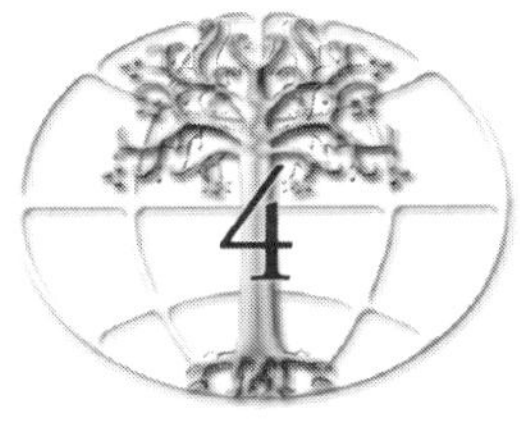

"It's a gift of being human to have the ability to heal – all you need is an open heart."
Kevin Farrow – founder of AcuEnergetics Australia.

Your First Session

What an incredible blessing it was to have the introduction I had into my contract. That a great friend very deliberately pushed me over the starting line, then gave me a good thrust in the back to ensure I went forward. I have never, and will never, forget what a gift that was.

Initially I became dependant on that, and on him. Perhaps it was habit that I expected him to guide me. Throughout our schooling we were taught, guided, and disciplined, by superiors, by teachers, and in that environment we learned, academically, at least. In that environment, they controlled the education, and we were content for them to control it. *This* learning environment, however, it was a whole new school of learning.

This environment demanded that I quickly recognize

that fact that my friend was my introduction, not my teacher. And thus, my first true conscious lesson in responsibility was discovered.

I was forced to realize that I walk alone. That this road, undiscovered and challenging, foreign and yet somehow recognizable, is mine alone. Just as yours is. Don't be frightened off by that. You will have people that, as is appropriate, will walk beside you, even hold your hand for a while. But ultimately the journey and the responsibility is yours.

It takes real emotional maturity to accept that, doesn't it? To accept that you are responsible. Especially in a world where society attempts to lay blame everywhere and anywhere else, rather than admit misgivings. Perhaps that is why a significant percentage of people that do come in my door, seeking to step into their journey, are over a certain age; usually in their mid forties. Maybe it takes a certain level of life experience, a developing of wisdom, lending them that emotional maturity and strength to venture forward in this way.

For me the lessons ran hard and fast from the beginning. The first few weeks in adjustment were very, *very* hard. Within me was a blur of change and adaptation and a battle within for acceptance. This was made all the more difficult when I went into a very deep depression. The kind of depression where you're picking out the tree to run your car into. I know now, as my education has continued and I am still learning, why I went mentally, consciously where I did. But at the time it felt shocking, the angst almost unbearable; and the answers were not forthcoming.

The first few months weren't a whole lot easier. These frequencies never stopped. The instruction manual was within, but in my infancy I could not access it. I had to grow first. I would go to bed, and instead of resting, in the dark of night the frequencies were amplified. All night my arms, shoulders and back would burn and buzz and tingle. I would close my eyes and try to rest, only to be assaulted by a barrage of color and light beneath my closed eyelids.

And clients were coming! People I would never have met in my once "normal" life were coming to me, *me*, for healings.

Worse, there were still no answers anyone could, or would, give me. Believe me I read, searched, asked, begged, rang, dropped by, prayed, you name it. The quest to understand not just the "why", which would be all about me, but the "how" this was happening, was underway and with each question answered, the list of questions grew.

Regardless, the lessons were lessons nonetheless. From them came recognition, education, even a little wisdom I'd like to think, but most importantly came the explanation and introduction for you. And you don't need to go through the brutality that I did, because I did it for you. You get to skip that (You can thank me later, when you know a little more).

Each lesson usually came in the form of a client experience. Client sessions remain to this day my primary classroom. Of course there are other circumstances in which I learn, but that is where most of your lessons will come from too: *my* client sessions!

The evolution of this form of healing has been extraordinary. It's involved some really harsh moments, blatant deceptions and personal injury, as well as all the exemplary wonder of it all. There really is balance in everything. Throughout all of it, I have continued with these sessions. And now, I ask anyone who works with me to hold me to my promise, that, come what may, I will always continue to do private healing sessions. For therein lies the genuine education.

What I consider "normal" in life these days I would have scoffed at a few years ago.

From the outset I want to address what's happening during a healing session. Or at least address, at this stage, the stuff we know. I'll get onto the "stuff we're pretty sure of" later. From all perspectives, dimensions and sensations I can address it from, let's talk about these "miraculous" healing sessions.

This is, absolutely, a cross-over between the spiritual and the physical; big time! A lifting of the veil, if you will. People report unique and very detailed descriptions of the events of a journey, or spiritual entity or experience, every time.

These frequencies in themselves are quite distinct and deliberately obvious for us to see. As palpable as they are in sensation, they will also make themselves visible whilst in operation. In the position of facilitator, you will clearly see and feel evidence that the client on which you are working is "in session".

I could go into detailed explanation here, or instead I could show it to you. I choose the latter. After all, as I read on my son's school teacher's blackboard:

Tell me, I'll forget
Show me, I'll remember
Involve me and I'll understand
Let me take your hand as you become involved…

Stuart's story encompasses all that is amazing in session.

I received the call from Stuart's wife just before Christmas. Stuart was riddled with cancer, and had been given four weeks to live three and a half weeks before they called me for a healing session. Going for the maximum miracle!

I went to them, as he was terribly ill and travelling would have exhausted him. When I arrived, several family members were hovering about a very thin, very yellow gentleman who happened to have his head in a bucket as he vomited. Stuart's cancer had originated in the liver and kidneys, and spread throughout his body over the last two years. They had tried all sorts of treatment and remedies and had been misled by another "healer", who by the sound of it, cashed in nicely. A friend of theirs that I had recently assisted had recommended me.

Throughout the sessions we underwent the family were present in increasing numbers. I know that some healers recommend against this. For me, I have no issue with it. I have nothing to hide, and as my experience has increased with this extraordinary gift I find that sometimes the healing isn't just for the person on the table. This particular case really demonstrated this point.

As I started the session, initially about the head, I had nothing…no feedback into my hands. The energy was moving through me, and strongly, but his body was offering no response. So I moved along his body, slowly, waiting for his body to start "talking". Nothing.

It has happened now with several cases, where a body has been chronically ill for some time, that it seems almost as though the body is just tired. Worn out from constant battle, it seems to need an injection of energy to initiate that "flow" again. Stuart's body was like this. It took about five or six minutes, using my eyes most of the time, to get his body to start responding so that I could feel the energy response. With my hands, I started at his feet and slowly worked up over the body.

Outside the birds had started making the racket as they often do. The birds near my regular rooms are used to it now, and usually just sit on the fence outside the window. But in a new environment, such as Stuart's home… Common birds, starlings, peaceful doves, were frantically and haphazardly flying just outside the windows, making a huge amount of noise. A couple got caught in the washing line, and a couple flew headlong into the windows, startling the family no end.

Lights started flashing about the ceiling, flicking on and off, not unlike fireflies, but faster. There were very distinct presence in the room, and it felt like a celebration. A large presence stood and seemed to cradle Stuart's head, and as long as it was there, I was unable to work around the head. Another stood at his right knee, and reappeared for all three sessions.

As we worked, Stuart had stopped breathing for a couple of minutes, and then with a huge gasp his entire body arched up off the table. And the birds outside stopped as though a switch had been thrown.

When someone this ill stops breathing for a short time, I admit it worries me. It's quite common in all clients, but remember Stuart was very ill. With Stuart, while I was busy indicating to family that it was all perfectly normal, nodding and smiling assuredly at them, my heart was pounding. I confess there were a couple of moments where I was about to start compressions on the heart, "Nothing to worry about! This is all part of the healing technique…"

The first session lasted for about an hour and a half. When Stuart opened his eyes his smile was blinding. Both of us had become aware during the session that a decision had to be made by him as to whether or not he wanted to stay. His body was tired but if he needed to stay, he could. He told me the man at his right knee was his father and had told him he had "come to take him home". And the large man at his head was the fifth guru, of the Sikh religion, Stuart's chosen religion.

For the first time in several weeks Stuart was able to eat and to speak. When he had closed his eyes prior to the session they were yellow with jaundice, and when he opened them they were white and clear.

I saw Stuart again the following day. Physically he was very, very tired, but he was most insistent that we continue. His body flowed richly with frequency, and this time the majority of the work was over his body, with the exception of the area around the heart and around his head. This time the large presence seemed to have his hands over Stuart's heart, and stood at his left side. This session was also well over an hour.

The movement around and about the area I was working was quite palpable. There was a swirling breeze about the treatment table, cool and somehow friendly. Stuart's little dog, so protective of his master, was sitting under the table. This poor little guy didn't know what to make of it, and you could see his dilemma whether or not to stick it out. Eventually it got too much for him and he raced through his doggy door outside. Unfortunately the birds were going berserk out there, and a matter of seconds later he tore back in again.

The light in the room, mostly in the upper half of the room, was like sunlight reflecting off water. Unusually for me, I could see colours around Stuart; a beautiful halo of light blue about his head, and a soft yellow about his chest.

Again the question was put to Stuart as to whether he would stay or not. He later recounted that this time his father said to him, "I have come to ease this pain, and take you home". When he opened his eyes they were clear and happy, and his smile again was wonderful. All of his pain had gone.

At this stage, fear got the best of me. I was pretty sure that he was going to die on the table. As usual what I was seeing at this end, was very, well, physical. Perhaps he would take off and decide not to come back. It's happened with many others, that where they were was so beautiful, they resented your tap on the shoulder. So a frantic exchange of email began between myself and my support crew of friends and teachers. "He's gonna die! He's gonna die on the table! Can I refuse to go back?!" One friend, Eric, a businessman, being sensible and concise and just a tad humorous, said to me, "Has he signed a disclaimer?"

After this second session, I recommended that we leave Stuart's body to heal for at least a day before I returned. When I did return and he saw me, tears streamed down his face. Stuart was in a lot of pain, had lost his ability to speak again, and was clearly distressed. We went to work immediately, and again the session was long. Again, there was a light bluish haze about his head as I worked, and this time it became clear the decision he had made...

When he opened his eyes, again they were clear, and he nodded his head. He was still in pain around his kidneys, so I did a little more hands-on work for him. Then he said he was tired and I helped him to his bed. Up until now Stuart had refused to take any pain relief, so we discussed budgeting (he was a successful businessman), and I suggested he use his energy for his family rather than tolerating pain. His wife phoned his oncologist, and they were to go to the hospital later that day. We spoke a little more, and then I said farewell and left.

Thiry six hours later the phone rang. It was Stuart's wife. They had gone to the hospital to undergo some tests for the pain relief, and while they were there the doctors had done an ultrasound of the liver and kidneys. There was no cancer to be found. They repeated the tests, and added a few to the list, and again there was *no trace of the cancer.* They kept Stuart in overnight, as they wanted to delve further, but he was exhausted.

The following morning his family went in and found him sitting up and chatting. He was in no pain, although clearly very tired. He spoke to his family, his wife and each of his children, kissed them all, closed his eyes and simply stopped. Stuart died. Just quietly, painlessly, slipped away. The doctors were nearly in tears when the family refused to let them do an autopsy.

His wife had called me, as they wanted me to attend the funeral. Hundreds attended this funeral, and when I entered I stood toward the back out of respect, somewhat conspicuous as the tall, blonde, pregnant woman who hadn't thought to cover her hair! Stuart's family stood by the open casket. His eldest son looked up and saw me and started to edge his way through the crowd toward me. I braced myself for the "Some healer you are!" As he reached me, he silently took my hand

and led me back through the crowd to the casket. When I looked in at Stuart, placing a flower upon his heart, I noticed that they had placed a light blue turban on his head, as I had seen in his sessions. I looked up at his children, his wife, all smiling through the tears cascading down their cheeks.

In the week that I spent with Stuart and his family I saw a huge transition, from fear and denial of an impending death, to a comfortable acceptance and transition into it, for all of them. Of course they miss him. But a monumental shift occurred *for all of them* as Stuart was able to die comfortably.

I am aware that this particular story isn't the greatest endorsement for healing. After all, he died. He was free of cancer, and still he died. Throughout the week that I knew him, Stuart and I knew that he had a choice. He didn't have to leave. This was his choice. It also taught me that sometimes death *is* the healing. Louder than ever we see that death is no "ending".

Stuart went Home. His family continued. Yet, in that same week, an amazing transition occurred for each of his family and friends. The first meeting I had with them, they were terrified Stuart might die, and desperate to halt it. They weren't in denial, but they so desperately wanted to be. At his funeral, only a week later, they were not happy to farewell him, but they were at peace with the journey. Each of them, in lesson during Stuart's dying, had undergone a healing all their own.

Stuart was a great man who came from the heart, and even in his death was so generous that he gave to us this entire beautiful, all encompassing lesson.

In session, the experience is always unique. It has to be, because each of us is unique. There is always a healing, although it is not always what you may desire. That being said, it's unusual if someone comes to you with cancer, or AIDS, or MS, and that is not the body's priority to heal. It does happen, but rarely.

In session there is always learning, intrinsically and, quite often, introspectively. And often, there is a spiritual experience of such magnitude that the physical response is often secondary in the client's mind. People open their eyes and more often than not start to tell you that they spoke to someone, or that they saw someone or some place, smelt an exquisite fragrance, and many other experiences. Only later do they say, "All my pain is gone!" or notice the physical response to the session.

In some sessions, the physical response is instant. A man paralysed down his right side by a stroke, unable to move arm or leg and had lost the ability to speak, opened his eyes after the session and said, quite clearly, "I don't feel any different." He then lifted his right arm, and rubbed his eye as he turned to his wife. "No, I don't feel a thing." Unlike him, she was speechless.

Should you choose to work in this form of healing, whatever modality or profession you are in or have experienced, I guarantee these sessions will be unprecedented for you. I'm not saying it's better, or that it has "superseded" anything or anyone. But it *is* unprecedented in our time. It is majestic in presence, and awesome in response.

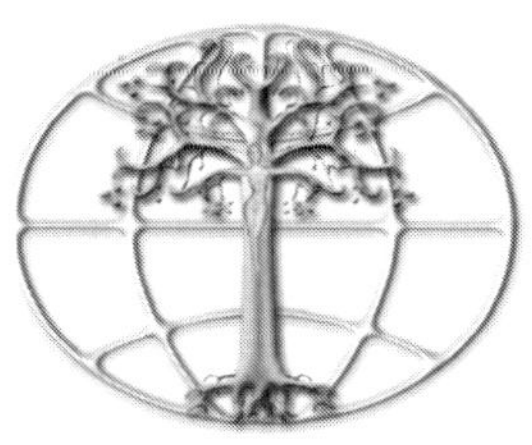

Individual Evolution

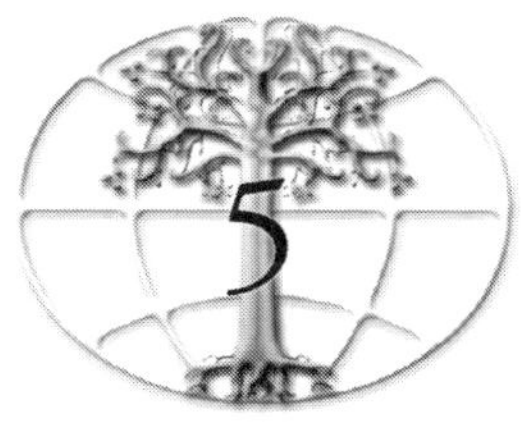

"The purpose of life is to discover life within life… reconnecting with that divinity ever present, but hiding within." ***Kryon***

And so it began…

You're fairly well versed now about my very first day in the realm of this gift. An astonishing day, to say the least. You would have thought I'd take a day or two off to adjust and recover from the initial thrust off the edge and into the abyss, but no.

People started arriving at my door, seeking healing. People I never would have met in this life approached the front door of our house, looking apprehensive yet determined, and say, "Are you that healing lady?" or "Are you that lady that helps people?" or simply "I have cancer." One or two a day would show up, at first. Then someone's mother had arthritis, someone's nephew had ADHD, someone's grandmother had Alzheimer's, and people would come. Our home phone became more of a call centre, our living room a makeshift healing centre.

It became clear that I needed another treatment table. I did have a treatment table, it was only Lynn who had been forced to lie upon the dining room table, and I needed a table that could travel. It was easier, as I was starting out, to go and see people rather than have them come to me. Travelling to see clients was best, particularly when the client was suffering chronic illness, or in the latter stages of terminal disease. I found it worked better to go to them if it was reasonable.

Not wanting to challenge myself too much financially, I perused the classified section of the Melbourne Trading Post, trying to pick up something decent, second-hand. They should make this sort of shopping a blood sport. The competition for anything decent is fierce. So first thing on the day the paper came out I made several calls answering any ads that looked okay, only to be told "I'm sorry, it's gone," or "I'm sorry, it's sold." I heard it again and again. On one of these calls I went to an answering service.

That night, I was pretty much decided that I would save myself the grief and buy a new table when the phone rang. A young woman, Jenny, said to me, "Hi, are you looking for a treatment table?"

She didn't want to deal with the harassing, so she had let the all of them go onto her answering machine until it maxed out. When she got home from work, she listened to all the messages until she heard mine, the eleventh, and called me. She thought I sounded 'nice'.

Jenny asked me what I wanted the table for and when I told her, she became very excited.

"You're a spiritual healer?" She gasped.

"Well, no not quite…"

"But a kind of spiritual healer, right; I mean you use the spirits to heal, yes?"

"Sort of, but..."

"Oh my God! I had a clairvoyant reading last week and

she told me to find you! She told me to find you! When I heard your voice, I didn't listen to any other messages. I called you! I found you!"

After a stunned silence came my fragile reply, "Okay."

The table sounded great, brand new, never been used, and we made arrangements for me to do a healing session on her when I went to pick it up.

Jenny had a hideous experience with recreational drugs about twelve months prior to our meeting. Initially, she had suffered a form of psychosis where she had left her body involuntarily and couldn't get back into it, try as she continually did, for more than twelve hours. Her friends had her rushed to the hospital, where over the following several days she went between high degrees of terror, paranoia and depression, all the while consistently fighting suicidal thought patterns. These attacks gradually decreased over the next few months. But on that fateful day when I met this lovely girl, Jenny was still regularly having severe anxiety attacks, worthy of hospitalization.

Prior to this unfortunate event, Jenny had had a successful career and life, on the whole, but was now reclusive and unable to work. She was beautiful, popular and talented, and her family despaired at her situation. Over the past twelve months Jenny had spent more than fifty thousand dollars on anything that could help her, from conventional medicine to the highly unconventional, and even a trip to Disneyland (really, if anything can cheer you up Disneyland can).

When I arrived I was greeted by two of the most exquisite Dobermans, clearly trained to protect her. She was utterly delighted when, after only a couple of minutes, the dogs gave me the ultimate canine compliment and sat on my feet.

I tried out my new table (exactly what I wanted). It was a fairly long session. Oddly her dogs had been barking out in the yard, but throughout the session they fell silent. Jenny was frightened because of what the previous year had been like, and initially had trouble just letting go. She later told me that she had opened her eyes and looked at me, and though I somehow looked different, she knew it was me. And all of a sudden she knew she was *safe*. Soon after that moment she had quite the journey. At the time Jenny had a heavy cold and her nose was blocked, but throughout most of it she was inhaling, sniffing deeply.

When she awoke she spoke of the most exquisite smell, she "couldn't get enough of it", and of a woman with long, dark hair picking white flowers in a beautiful garden. She claimed, as several people have, that she couldn't begin to describe the smell, it was "unlike anything I've ever smelt before". The entire time she had felt a little warm weight on her chest. The moment I touched her shoulder, indicating the session was over, the dogs starting barking to come into the house again. She looked up at me, smiled, and was plainly a different woman…

When she got off the table she seemed to move as though she was no longer carrying a physical burden. She moved as though buoyant and was all smiles and, I guess, joyous. We sat at her kitchen table while she told me about the session, laughing and basking in her new light.

She refused any money for the table.

Two weeks later she rang. Life had been testing her out and she'd had some stressful situations arise. Jenny claimed any one of the situations would have hospitalized her in the past, let alone what all of them together would have done, but she handled them with confidence, and as she put it, "not an ounce of fear!" In reaction to these circumstances, she'd had not so much as a brief shortness of breath. She had taken a job managing a huge retail store and was really enjoying it. She no longer feared sleep and often felt as though there was someone with her. Work colleagues, family and friends could not believe the difference in her, often asking her to 'come down off that cloud you're on.' Jenny had found what many of us seek: *relief.*

I had been practicing for several weeks when I met Jenny. Her session, what happened from her perspective and from mine was rich in lesson and enveloped as such. What had occurred for Jenny within the two weeks that followed showed me that there was far more that I needed to embrace in order for this work to progress.

The third night after I had met and worked on Jenny, I had yet another restless night where my upper back, arms and hands had burned and buzzed all night. When I awoke and went to the kitchen to get the day started for the clan, I reached for a cup and noticed the palms of my hands felt kind of numb. As you do, without thinking, I flipped my hand over to look at my palm on my left hand, and was met with one of the most extraordinary sights;

My palms were imprinted with a geometrically precise pattern made up of hundreds and hundreds of dots like someone had been pushing a fine pen tip into the flesh of my hands. My left palm was completely covered in these incredible patterns and on down past my wrist, my right was about seventy percent covered with a solid patch completely bare.

I reeled backwards physically when I first looked at my hand, apparently trying to get away from it. I was leaning against the kitchen wall, my hands out in front of me, just gaping at them. I must have looked pretty distressed because Andrew came in saying "What is it? What's wrong?" I showed him.

He voiced what I couldn't at the time, "What the hell…?"

He looked at me, "Do they hurt?"

I shook my head.

"How did you do it?"

I looked at him, "How *would* I do it?!"

"You just woke up with it?"

I nodded. Then I said something weird, "We should do

a drawing of them. I should try to draw these patterns. People need to know about them."

This was weird because, in this day and age, why wouldn't you take a photo? Andrew is a professional computer nerd, and we had every camera gadget you can imagine. An ink print of them would have been more high tech than "drawing" them, and certainly more believable in evidence. Andrew was holding my forearms (not being game to hold my actual hands) and we were both staring at my hands. Then he looked up at me, and in his gaze for the first time I could see he was wondering who I was. Of course, I was too. It was the first time I felt utterly alone in this.

Over several hours they gradually faded, and finally they went away. I only had them that once. And no, I have no bloody idea why. You can imagine the theories: an initiation of some sort (alien, I'm sure), an alien abduction, holy image, etc. It was probably more likely that Spirit had discovered I was a tad dogmatic in this, so I needed a really obvious sign. You know; if you can't coax them forward, push them.

Over the following twelve months I would see several clients who, when they opened their eyes after the session, would marvel at the incredibly detailed and intricate geometric patterns on the ceiling.

"My goodness the detail on your ceiling is incredible! It must have taken you ages to paint."

The ceiling, of course, was plain white. Two claimed these patterns were the same as the structure of a cathedral ceiling in Europe. Only twice did I think to show any of these people the hand patterns, and both times they were the same as what they saw on the ceiling.

And it didn't change what I was experiencing as I facilitated healing sessions (rest assured strange hand patterns are not essential). It did, once again, alter the direction of the path I was on a little. And again I had to recognize the need to look within in order to understand more, to listen. And still people kept coming, and I kept listening and playing and learning.

When I was twelve, I put my name in a barrel to win a pony. Without ever really even thinking about it, before I'd even put my name in the barrel, I knew that the pony was mine. There was a certainty that I can still feel today. A few days after I put my name in, much to my father's horror, a little Shetland pony called Lightening, moved to our property amid the thoroughbreds and quarter horses we already had.

My friend had shown me the gift that was within, even nurtured a detailed introduction with it, and he had suggested that I go to Los Angeles to learn a version of the axiatonal procedure he had done on me: the two day procedure that was the key to my own explosion into this. At the time he suggested it, it seemed an utter impossibility: I had two babies, one with severe disabilities, and financially it was a struggle... so of course, a few weeks later I was in L.A.

To his credit, my husband had pushed me to go to L.A. He knew it was important that I continue. In the week before I was due to fly out, however, trauma reared its ugly head: my beautiful sister-in-law, Simone, died suddenly and tragically. All of the arrangements had to be made. My son was fulltime in a wheelchair and wearing a broomstick plaster on both of his legs after some radical orthopaedic surgery. My little girl had only just been weaned from the breast.

Life can be like that, can't it? Just when you decide to set a goal, or commit to something, Life throws a few hurdles at you just to make sure you're serious. Not being a victim by nature, I just get on with the business of dealing with it all. And it was quite incredible how it all fell into place in the eleventh hour, so I could get on the plane and go. I took it as confirmation. And that is what this trip to L.A was all about…confirmation.

Despite what appeared to be insurmountable hurdles, I had that same certainty that I had had about the pony; an unquestionable certainty that I would be in L.A. As objective onlooker, I watched, as it all fell into place, and even when I stepped off the plane at LAX, it was in the knowledge that it was meant to be, rather than wonder at the synchronicity.

I couldn't wait to get there. I had hundreds of questions. What's more, this was considered an advanced process, and I had great hopes of meeting practitioners who were doing what I was doing, experiencing what I was experiencing (despite what little I knew consciously), and meeting people of like mind and life changing shift!

One of the greatest gifts of this journey was Larry. An old and very dear friend of Savannah's, he was another of those warm and beautiful living guides that enter your life and Larry was under her instructions to take care of me. And that is exactly what he did. Larry is a huge, warm, intelligent man, with the loyalty of a Labrador and the courage of a lion. He is fabulous. We were instant friends, and rapidly he became my guardian. I had five days in L.A, and he made sure I saw everything an Aussie girl should, despite the fact that most of my time was taken up with the course.

In one night we went down Santa Monica Boulevard, up Sunset, down Melrose, and then walked the stars on Hollywood Boulevard. I would be hungry and he would find whatever food I asked for. More than that I would be overwhelmed, and he would level me out. And he has the best laugh; honest, rich and contagious.

Larry attended the course with me. So, yes, we did laugh a lot. It became clear that my anticipations were, again, utterly incorrect. My hopes of meeting amazing and learned practitioners left me, for the most part, terribly disappointed. I was to discover even more ego at play in this room than I had seen in that workshop in Melbourne. And it was no small room with 320 people and something like 80 massage tables. Surviving this workshop, especially the third day, was like surviving being cast adrift in a choppy ocean. The room was charged with a huge amount of frequency, as everyone was learning this procedure and it affected everything. You could see the changing energies in the room affecting everyone differently. People were riding the emotional rollercoaster that these frequencies can induce and riding it hard. It was exhausting to watch.

One minute a man would walk past and to my eyes he was hot! Very attractive, I'd say to Larry "Ooh, not bad Larry," and he'd say, "Mmm, not bad. I saw better last night." Five minutes later, after Larry's recounting the events of the previous night, the same man would go past again, and he appeared completely different! Larry would say, "Are you kidding me?" While all I could muster was a deflated and disappointed, "What happened to him?" It was fascinating.

Right from the outset, it was clear that I wasn't there to *learn* this procedure. Somehow, I already knew it. It just flowed through me fluidly, effortlessly, as if it was the most natural thing in the world for my body to do. It felt like a beautifully choreographed dance I'd always known. Going through the motions of this procedure for me was one of those exquisite moments in life when nothing else matters; all you know is bliss.

People were struggling to get their hands in the right position, to remember where the next line was, the next point, which direction their hand should be in, for this is not a simple procedure. Watching them and their very deliberate actions, you could almost hear the mind chatter of self doubt and of the pressure they were putting themselves under. These people, and their desire to be exceptional, were awesome. Well, okay, *some* of them were awesome. Others were there so that I could learn patience. Like a front row audience member I was able to watch as these people forced their own hands, and triggered what would be a few more steps forward in their journey to know themselves. A very deliberate decision, probably not consciously, that would take them closer to their own purpose. You have to love that, "reconnecting with that divinity, ever present, but hiding within."

The group was divided into sections for the purpose of teaching, and the group I was in would be called to work at the tables. I would saunter over to the nearest table ready to start. Another group would be called to lie on the tables to be practiced upon, and the table I was at would be mobbed by seven, eight, ten people! So I would think, "This table's popular. I'll just go to another." And select another table, whereby, of course, again it would be mobbed!

Larry told me later that as he was standing in the crowd observing, he heard a group of people discussing me. One lady said, "Get that woman (me) to work on you. She's really powerful!" (Larry cracked many a joke about this.) And they went on to discuss whatever they had experienced while I had worked on them. I was oblivious to all of this. Sadly, and often to my own detriment, I usually am oblivious to stuff like that.

This experience in L.A. was the first of a series of concentrated acceleration periods (other than my introduction, of course) in my "healing" journey. And Larry was my guide. I don't think either of us was counting on that. It happens somewhat regularly that I find myself away from all that is familiar, for a relatively short time span, with one individual who plays the role of guardian and helps to keep my feet on the ground while occasionally throwing in some brutal honesty to boot (there is nothing like a good slap in the face when you're contentedly enveloped in your own denial!). On these compact and purposeful occasions a huge amount happens in a very tight space in time! Despite any hint of adversity, despite the person that would seek to do you injury being right next to you, magic keeps happening. L.A. was the first time I would see this sort of period, and the first of these intense lessons that I now cherish so.

So to my guardians; Savannah, Larry, Lynn, Chris,

Tanja, Helen, I say to each of you, know that you are recognized and appreciated for the enormous teachers and friends that you are.

What did I learn in LA? I learnt about me. That was really what everyone that "workshop" was doing: learning about themselves. It was the first place I really learnt that in order to go forward I would have to go within. It was time for me to recognize the contract that mapped out this life, and the role I'd agreed to play in it. When I had been told I "had a gift" for healing, I had scoffed. This, in the face of what I already had been driven to in life, as a physiologist, and yet I still denied it.

Just after I had returned to Australia, our financial manager came to our house for a meeting and asked me why I had had to go to L.A. so suddenly. Peter is as straight laced as they come – an accountant. I did my best to explain, activated his hand so he could feel it, and told him what I seen so far. Then I looked at him and said, "So… do you think I've lost my mind?"

He looked me straight in the eye, slowly shook his head in that "surely not" way, and answered, "If it were anyone else, Mel… but it's you." He looked at the hand I had just worked on, "My hand is still…this is incredible! You know my wife is having trouble with her eyes…"

There are few situations in life where I feel completely carefree. When I am dancing, I don't think at all, it just happens. It's fluid and completely free of any of life's complications for me. I have no concern for how I might look, or what others might think, or any of that incidental ineffectual rubbish. I just dance, truly revelling in it. This work is like that for me, too. It's fluid and free and belongs within me so that it just flows without. And that ecstatic unrestricted spiritual dance is as present as ever now as it was when I started. In fact, probably more so.

Each day I awaken wondering "what will be before me

today?", "What will I be privileged to see today?" I wake feeling grateful, regardless of what has happened in this life. I mean, you have to be, don't you? This is enormous! Genuinely awesome! And you and I have front row seats in the evolutionary opera. Please don't lose sight of that. Always be glad, be grateful that *this is you* and *this is your time.*

Gratitude. Each day I wake up and it's my first emotion of the day. It's hard not to smile, when I think of what may just happen on this day. But, perhaps even more importantly, in the privileged task I have, I have seen the most amazing things happen. Gratitude plays a big role in this, as it ideally should in all things. It keeps your ego in check by reminding you that you are not the healer, you are the instrument. You know in your own heart there is a greater plan at play here and how can you help but be grateful for your part, conduit healer? Walt Whitman said it beautifully,

"That the powerful play goes on, and you may contribute a verse."

I love walking this planet. Don't you? I love all the little wonders and all the divine experiences it is to be human. In this, as a facilitator, I know another carefree moment. I cherish that it is so easy to remember what is really important and regain an appropriate perspective even under the most stressful circumstances. By stepping with bare feet on dewy grass, or closing your eyes and feeling the warm breeze caress your skin, or closing your eyes and listening to the wind in the eucalypts which sounds remarkably like the ocean and in your mind you can be transported (I used this one quite a lot when I was in the Army).

When was the last time you really looked at the perfection in a single flower? Think about it now. Just a daisy, or an iris, or a rose… its colour, shape, how each petal seems measured in size and placement, the colours and hues. And with that perfection in mind, now think of the human body…its complexity, its symbiotic balance, and its perfect and unrivalled beauty. How each movement is the most complex orchestration internally, but outwardly is nothing more than a single step. I know I fell in love with the divine integration of physiology.

To know gratitude through recognizing the immense gift that is within your grasp, is a given. Of course we are grateful. But when was the last time you knew gratitude for the privilege of being here? Whatever your circumstances, wherever you are, it is no accident that you are here. And you still have choice on your side.

Remember, as you go forward on your road, just how great it is to walk this planet. Slow down occasionally and experience the perfection of the moment. For in doing so, you are creating more perfect moments.

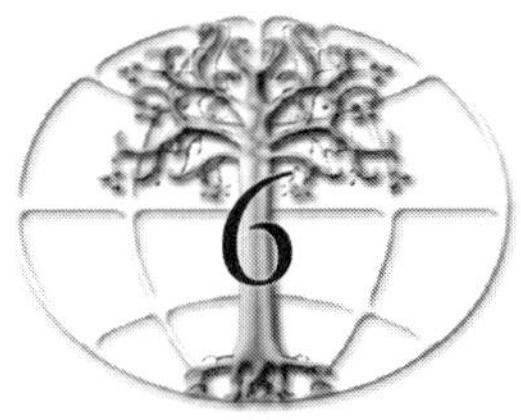

"Honour your body, which is your representative in this universe. Its magnificence is no accident. It is the framework through which your works must come; through which the spirit and the spirit within the spirit speaks. The flesh and the spirit are two phases of your actuality in space and time. Who ignores one, falls apart in shambles. So it is written..."
The Sacred Script of the Covenant / Ancient Sumari text

The Human Biology

The human body is an intricate and exquisite sculpture in balance.

When looking upon a human body it is both simple and complex. It is simple in its requirements, in its symmetry and balance, and in its obvious beauty. Complex when you start to investigate the intricacies; reduce the body to its chemical, cellular, molecular level, and all that it does, involuntarily, consciously unguided, brilliant in its mechanical ability to self balance and self distribute. Frankly, it will blow your mind! It is absolutely bloody incredible how human biology exists! Its magnificence really is no accident.

Simple and complex. It's all a matter of perspective really.

Isn't it always?

Now we all know we have different systems in the body, made up of varying essential organs, soft tissues, hard and soft muscles, skeleton, nervous system, brain, etc. The technical term for this is "parts". We all know this. Again, and perhaps it's the Indigo again breaking it down to its simplest form, but I want to simplify how you look at the amazing machine you walk around in (your body). The time has come to alter another predetermined paradigm.

The human body is a collective of cells, not a bunch of "parts". In order to address just *how* a body is healing from immersion in quantum bioenergetics, we need to adjust our primary perspective of it.

Recent discoveries have found evidence, an implication, that your entire biological cellular countenance is a community experience providing our consciousness with a vehicle for this life. All that exists is housed within the cellular memory, from the spiritual to the biological mechanics, and every cell feels everything and has an awareness of the whole. Each and every cell has a consciousness of the whole. Each one participates in the vibration of the complete human. *A community experience.*

We've talked of cellular memory, of spiritual memory, of life contracts and patterns, imprints and awakenings, so to think of cellular memory at the mundane biological level probably feels a little superficial, even inadequate. *Wrong.*

Instead of the anatomical systems we've learnt in Year Eight biology, and in the face of the healing facilitation we're addressing, let's separate the body into some elemental systems you may not have considered before.

Human biology consists more of an interchange, a synergetic relationship between our individual essence, our soul, interacting with our more subtle bodies (such as *axiatonals, meridians, chakras, energy systems*) and they in turn interact with our physical body.

These three elements of spirit or soul, energy anatomy, and the physical, are one; a weave of awareness, energies and matter that culminate into the vehicle in which we walk this planet: our body.

Everything you take in or do to this body of cells, every emotion and experience, affects each and every cell. There are some forms of medicine, founded in tradition and through generations of discovery, that have taken this into account for centuries. In its community awareness *each cell is aware of the whole*, and therefore *each cell represents the whole.* (In a few short chapters, you're about to palpably experience this first hand. You'll be amazed how much you already know, and how readily you can recognize it.) Every cell knows what every other cell is doing.

The body's ability to recover itself is extraordinary, for when in balance each cell can rejuvenate itself perfectly. Given it is put in the right environment. Your body only requires you to honour it with proper intake, environmental wisdom and maintenance, and it will do the rest. The body is designed in balance, to balance, and when enveloped in a remotely appropriate environment, thrives in its ability to recover and rebalance.

Already as I write I can feel the ether going a little murky with the mental groans going up in anticipation of what I am about to say. And yes, you are right.

Your body needs to be in balance. You need to respect and care for the body that in this life, is you. If your cells hold all that is you, and your body is a collaborative of that cellular community, then yes, that body is you.

I love sports, but no, I am not a fitness freak. I love an adventure, and having been very ill myself, I love to feel strong and physically capable, so I do keep my body active. If someone phones me and says "let's go white water kayaking or horse riding," I'm able to do it at the drop of a hat (provided I can get a baby sitter, that is). And I am grateful, whenever I am in such an environment and amazing things happen, that my body is capable of getting me into the right place at the right time.

I eat fairly well, but not brilliantly. I drink, although not often (enough). I don't sleep enough (must talk to the kids about that). I am an anatomical physiologist and I probably know more about trans-fatty acids, and the aspartame effect on the cellular membrane than the average person and *still* I find myself occasionally tearing bites out of a Quarter Pounder! Shocking, I know.

I live a real life. And I love walking this planet and living it. So when I inadvertently do damage to this body, I counter it as soon as I get the chance.

I do not stand in judgment of you, for I am in no worthy position to do so! I do not know how you live or what you do. But, all the same, I ask you to indulge me in my love of the divine biology we are, and allow me to share this concept with you…

Imagine that, when you came of age and got your license, a man from the licensing agency arrived on your doorstep, saying, "Congratulations! You now have your license and the responsibility to drive. What type of car would you like, then? You can have *any* car you like; any design or construction on the planet! Price is not a concern for you, it's free! The car is yours completely. So tell me, which car will you have?"

What would be going through your head now? What would your dream car be? What would it look like? Can you see it?

Imagine now that dream car being delivered to you, immaculate and ready for action. As you sign for the delivery the gentleman continued,

"Enjoy your vehicle, then. Although…" he pauses and looks at you, "Do remember that this is the only car you will own in this lifetime. The only car. *Nobody gets a second car.*"

How would you treat this car? How would you drive it? Would you put in the discounted fuel, stretch it with a little artificial additive to get a few extra miles? Or would you put in the extra, extra, high octane, premium deluxe fuel? Do you think you'd check the oil and the water levels regularly? If it wasn't running quite right, would you just leave it or would you have it at the mechanic ASAP? How *would* you treat that car? Because this is the only car you're getting. And sadly the car cannot self rejuvenate. It is a given that one day the car will stop. You want to make the ride up until that moment as good as you can.

Don't plan on getting a second body. Not in this lifetime anyway.

The human body can, put in the right environment, rejuvenate itself. Phew! Your cells have the potential within, to recover and re-balance the human biology, as no medicine can hope to. For medicine itself, while often essential in the process, is more instrumental on the road to the balanced environment.

Another issue is at hand here too. As a healing facilitator you need to lead by example. I'm not talking about physical appearances here, I'm talking about wellness; Whole system balance. In order to balance, you really need to be in balance yourself. Primarily in this chapter I am referring to the physical, but this also applies emotionally, mentally, in your mind set and the thought patterns you allow. For now let's keep it to the biology.

Healing is a system of balance. Healers don't heal, they balance. Be honest with yourself here. Do you really believe that if you're out partying all night, binge drinking, snorting a little cocaine, eating rubbish, and clearly being generally unhealthy, that you will be of any value to your clients? If you're not in balance, how will you create balance for the person that asked for your help?

You don't need to become a vegan, or schedule yourself

for colonic irrigation. Let's not get extreme here, especially if I have to join in. My advice as a physiologist and as a human is to get your body to a *state of comfort.* This state of comfort is quite easy to recognize.

The body has some nicely obvious signs when you're in balance: you won't feel ill, you're not in pain, and if you climb a few stairs you won't pass out. If any of these things show themselves, general illness, pain, or some sort of cardio vascular failure, then *quickly* find someone who can put you into a more balanced environment.

Am I being sardonic? I'm afraid so. While I haven't addressed it yet, I'm not ignoring those of you that currently live with a chronic health issue, disease or permanent injury. I know that what is "normal" for you, with regard to a "state of comfort", is probably quite different from those living without serious disease, illness or injury. As "normal" as what my life is like since this quantum healing thing showed itself.

Regardless, please understand the importance of balance in you first, no matter what your life circumstance. Take care of yourself first. I know in the society that I have been raised in that this may sound incredibly selfish. It's not. The intent of one will always affect the many. To honour yourself first, is to honour those around you, too.

I mentioned earlier that in my family I am the centre of our house. If my attitude goes to hell, so does the rest of the household. You've heard it before: *"If Momma ain't happy, ain't nobody happy."* If you are in the right place in your mind, your health, your thinking, your heart, those around you cannot help but feel the effects too. Take care of you.

Whilst in Infantry, during my time in the army, we would physically push ourselves well beyond the reasonable limits, occasionally to our own detriment. There were times out in the field when the blisters on your feet were so bad that they had to be directly injected with Betadine (ouch) each day and yet we would carry on. After all you didn't want to be perceived as a wimp.

I had the privilege of working with some individuals from the commando corps who I expected to be extra tough, but was surprised to also find them extra smart. If the smallest physical injury came to light it was dealt with immediately. They promptly took the time to point out the value of addressing a minor injury, before it became major. You were considered stupid to do otherwise. After all, you don't want to be perceived as an idiot. The job that I was in was a responsible job, and to compromise that through some farcical bravado was counter-productive.

Balance you first. Then, in balance, you can be the better person you know yourself to be. In balance you can become the person you know yourself to be, now. Every day, be that person. Share with us the amazing you, so that we, too, can learn balance.

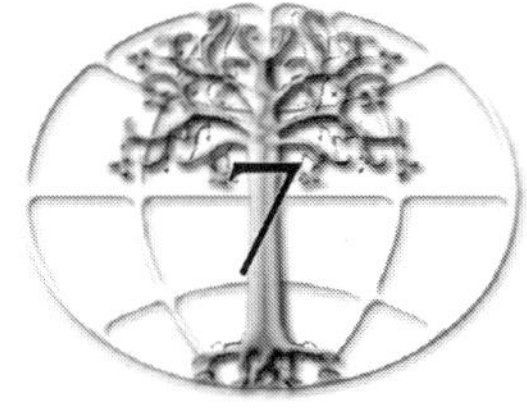

"As Below, so Above; And as Above, so Below.
With this knowledge alone you may work miracles."
Translation of the Emerald Tablet by Fulcanelli

Initiation turns into education

This incredible journey, like a reel of unravelling ribbon, continued to rapidly unfold; miraculous and enormously colourful, it wound itself in and out of lesson after lesson. Each client that walked in the door, would show me, or teach me something new. The speed at which these lessons were coming at me was astounding. Really, there were times when I thought; surely they would give me a break; time just to process and rest! But instead, there was an ever present pressure and drive pushing me onward, telling me to get on with the work. This time, unlike when I was ill and studying, I wasn't actually pressuring myself. This pressure, or "enthusiastic encouragement", was extrinsic and very much not of this world. (No, not aliens. C'mon, I thought we were over this!)

Rather than give me a break, in scaling this cliff-like

learning curve, I was given a gift in the form of an individual. As each stage progressed, each lesson or shift unfolded, I would be handed the gift of a friend, human, that could relate, and would help me to comprehend a little more. Someone to bounce everything off, sometimes they were people I met just once, sometimes a client would become more, sometimes they were people I already knew who had been waiting in the wings ready to play their role. And of course, there was Andrew, playing one of the most prominent roles of all. Great gifts came in the form of these people.

I received a call from a personal assistant requesting a healing session for her boss, a psychiatrist. Apparently her boss had suffered a fall, and amongst other lesser injuries had fractured her pelvis. She had recovered sufficiently from the pelvic injury to be back at work, but was still having pain.

Trying to schedule this client's session was a trial. She was clearly a very busy psychiatrist, but more than that, was absolutely insistent that I come to her rooms to do her session. To her credit, she got the better of me, and I found myself smiling ironically as I walked in the front gate of a beautiful home in the inner suburbs of Melbourne. It all became a little clearer, and even more intriguing, when I met her.

Merrill was eighty-six years old and still working full time as a clinical psychiatrist, lecturing at universities and conferences, and very sharp witted. She was just fabulous! She had extraordinary energy in her language and her activities, but her frustration was evident at what she felt was her body's betrayal of her. Her body was showing its age, especially after the recent accident that had caused the pelvic injury. Merrill also had a kyphosis in her upper back (a front to back curvature of her spine, a "c" shape), and a scoliosis (an "s" shaped, side to side curvature of her spine) that caused the pelvis to reside on a slight angle.

Her house was very much her home. On each wall of her house, which encompassed her professional rooms, were floor to ceiling bookshelves, interrupted by a compulsory window here and there, and what an exquisite library it was! I love books. I was in heaven. Even now, remembering them, I cannot help smiling at the beautiful, richly bound volumes that filled those shelves. One of my favourites, included amongst the many extraordinary titles, was Merrill's own Thesis, completed at the age of 76, which seemed directly related to the work I was doing!

Having had to go to her, I had gone in the early evening outside my usual hours. I think I made it home around 2am! We talked for ages, about her work, about mine, about the supposed "inactive" DNA junk, and cellular renewal (Merrill being more interested in brain function, chemical alteration, etc). She told me anonymous stories of some of the challenges past clients had presented her, (including a priest who didn't believe in Jesus! He *was* having trouble.)

Eventually, we got to her healing session. Her home, rich in history, experience and life, was an amazing environment in which to conduct a session. Full of memory, the activity in the room while I worked was almost overwhelming for me. Honestly, had I not spent the time with her that I had, and gained the assurance of the environment as I had, I don't think I could have stayed. At that time, fear could have won.

In terms of time taken, it was fairly average; a little over thirty minutes. Going into a session knowing the injury or ailment that has caused the person to call you isn't always an asset. In this case I found myself wondering why I was drawn to what appeared to feel like her spine when I knew the injury, and not a small one, was in her pelvis. Regardless, the intrinsic knowledge within, was telling me that I was not in charge here, meaning that I was to "listen" to the signals I'm given, and work where I'm lead to work. This body had been around a while too, so it wasn't far fetched that an age of eighty-six, minor bodily ailments would be present. Although I still recall the frustration I felt at the time, for she so much wanted the pelvic injury to be addressed.

As I worked around her, she was physically shifting and jerking a little, and it was clear most of the involuntary spasm was along the spine. Her legs would twitch a little, and her shoulders shifted only once or twice, but around her torso particularly the twitches and movement seemed constant.

The session finished and I touched her shoulder. She opened her eyes, smiled at me quietly, and then announced, "My whole back aches. What did you do?"

She tried to sit up, but "something felt different" and she didn't seem able to move as she had before. I assisted her in transitioning to a sitting position, thinking to myself, "This is where the physiologist comes in really handy." Then I looked at her.

Merrill was sitting differently. She was sitting straight, and tall. Her head was held at a new angle, the neck more upright, the shoulders back…then I realized her entire upper back had been pushed inward, back to what would be the ideal anatomical position. The forward curvature of the spine and hence the jutting angle of the neck and head, the kyphosis, was gone! I stared at her in wonder, as she said, "I feel a little off balance. Hmmm. Something is different here" then, with a smile, "Oh, Melissa! I have no pain at all. The pain in my hips is gone!" It seemed the pelvic injury was addressed, (Oh me of little faith!)

I was congratulating her on her fine work, at healing herself, while I again assisted her to stand up off the table. In the process of standing up she stamped her foot into the floor abruptly, like she had missed a step. Actually it was more like there was a step that she was unaware of. Merrill giggled, self conscious at her own instability, as she continued to tell me she felt "different", and was free of pain. I suggested she walk a little, see how the new hips worked.

As she walked away from me it was clear that even more had happened. Her pelvis was straight! No wonder her foot stamped into the floor, her leg would have felt longer. Her gait was completely altered, so her walking must have felt very strange to her! So much so that she turned to me and said,

"You know I really must get this floor re-stumped. It feels so terribly unstable, undulating underfoot! Oh… my whole back is aching."

When I had arrived, the scoliosis in her spine, the S like curvature, was plain to see. Now, after her session, it wasn't. I couldn't resist…

"Merrill, would you mind if I have a look at your back? Maybe I can see something that could help the ache."

Can you believe it? Her spine was dead straight!

Merrill stood against the wall and we measured her height. She had grown more than two inches in forty five minutes!

Of course her back was aching! More than seventy years of walking around in a certain way, the spine a certain shape, and hence the body adapting to it, a sudden straightening was bound to cause a few aches and pains for the rest of the body. No doubt all sorts of muscles and connective tissues were registering formal complaints with the brain.

I ended up calling in a fabulously instinctive masseur, Chris Warren, and together we worked with her for a few months to help her body adapt. The aches soon abated. Out of curiosity, we measured her height again, a couple of months after the initial session, and this time it was closer to three inches more than her original height.

I had known Chris Warren for a number of years. We had become great friends almost instantly. The kind of friend where you sit down for a coffee and eleven hours later your husband rings and says "Where are you? It's been 12 hours!" It is a true and enduring friendship.

When I called him, regarding Merrill, I hadn't had the chance to tell him what I was now doing. The healings, I mean. When I first met Chris, it was as a client back in the good old physiologist days, and I had I helped him to rehabilitate an injury. As happens in life, we hadn't seen a lot of each other in the past two years. I had had Jack, and all the drama that came with him, and Chris had been overseas, and when returned, was chronically ill for some months. That experience for Chris had changed his path, hence the extraordinary masseur he had become.

When he first came to work on Merrill, I did a quick session on her first. I had briefly explained to him what I now did, but evidently not enough. Chris sat on a sofa as I worked, quietly watching, long, lanky and relaxed. I got on with the session, not really even noticing him, until I passed by.

Chris was sitting upright gripping the edge of the sofa with both hands, and sweating profusely. As I wandered by, he looked up at me and started silently mouthing frantically, which I casually ignored and continued to pass by, hiding my smile.

Merrill's session ended, and Chris was forced to shroud himself in professionalism, so all he could say calmly and slowly was "That was powerful, wasn't it? Mel? Wasn't it?" But his eyes were saying "What the…?!" Merrill was having trouble relaxing as Chris worked on her, so I offered to quietly "zap" while he worked. Chris was brave and did his best to tolerate it, but eventually he begged me to stop. I confess I had been focused on Merrill, and it was only when Chris spoke up and I looked at the sweat pouring off him, and the shake in his hand, I recognized he too was getting the full brunt of Merrill's session!

Soon after we finished the session we left. You can imagine his reaction out on the street. You would have thought he'd just bungee jumped. He had the high-pitched, rapid banter that only a massive adrenaline rush can really bring on. I couldn't get a word in, which is saying a lot!

I tried to explain. (I'm still trying!). He had hundreds of questions, including "How on earth did you straighten out that woman's spine?" I offered him a session to experience it himself, to which he said, "Okay! Let's go!" It was 11pm. I had to get home. Chris' response was "That's okay. We'll go to your house." Oh, great!

Who would have thought? Yet another amazing shift forward.

We walked in the front door, and Andrew was immediately accosted by Adrenaline Chris and his verbal barrage. I set up the room while Andrew's eardrums took a high pitched beating.

The beauty for me, of this first session on Chris was that Andrew was able to witness it. It had been some time since he had seen me facilitate a healing session. Also being great friends with Chris, he sat in and watched. I don't know who was more fun to watch; Chris or Andrew.

In session Chris took off rapidly, not surprisingly considering the recent exposure he had had at Merrill's session. His physical reaction at this end was big; his entire lanky body was shuddering from head to foot, his breathing would stop and start (all normal). His arms moved slowly outward, laterally, from his body, and off the table so that they were perpendicular to his body and there they stayed. Then Chris' upper body arched up and away from the table. I'd seen this sort of response before and knew that this was only the beginning, so I started to alter the flow of frequencies through myself, the instrument, so that Chris wouldn't be distracted, or feel self conscious, about this involuntary physical response.

For the sake of the client's experience and to the best of their ability, you want the client to "let go"; to stop the mind chatter, and allow themselves to go with the frequency flow. You've heard of "mind over matter"? This is "mind over chatter". Not always easy, but the memory of the experience during their session, at a conscious level, is far clearer if they are able to let go. The involuntary physical reactions, particularly muscle spasms, and the larger gross motor movements, are distracting because, understandably, the individual can feel quite self conscious in front of the facilitator.

(*For the Healers out there: I know what you're thinking. No, this doesn't interfere with the client's experience. In fact it appears to enhance it as was the intention. I will explain more about this instrumental element, further ahead.*)

His body surrendered and relaxed a little more, but his physical reactions, eyes flickering, head movement, etc, were still going wild. I turned to smile at Andrew, only to find Andrew's jaw was on the floor and eyes wide with astonishment. He silently pointed at Chris's elevated upper body and his vibrating solar plexus. I turned back to Chris to find his eyes had involuntarily opened the pupils slightly askew from one another, and trying to find me. I kept working about the table, away from the body, not actually on Chris.

Chris's mouth started working but no sound was uttered. I thought to myself, "Here we go. He's going to channel." I looked down to see Andrew trying to move silently forward, clearly wanting to hear what Chris was saying. I started hoping Chris would channel just to see what Andrew would do! I know the first time I heard someone channel while on my table, I only just stopped myself from bolting out the door. (Only the fact that the person had paid me for his session kept me there at the time!)

I changed my approach, again subtly altering the application, and Chris's mouth stopped, his eyes closed, and his body went quiet again. But you could feel something brewing, "the calm before the storm" so to speak. Beads of sweat dotted his forehead, and he started his full body shudder again. I thought that was probably enough for a first timer, so I gently touched his shoulder.

He instantly opened his eyes, smiled for a while, said, "Mel" before the tears started to flow. This isn't unusual, as a response, but it's never really for the same reasons. There does seem to be an overwhelming beauty that although not always consciously remembered, is embraced deep within. The tears are a basic, if not crude, release in the face of such beauty. However, everyone's experience, everyone's journey is unique.

At the end of the session, when I touch someone on the shoulder, I don't tap them as such; I place my hand around their shoulder. I sort of embrace them in a small way and stay there for a few moments until I see that they're back again. I absolutely recognize the magnitude of what these people experience, and in this small way, I try to embrace and secure them as they return and open their eyes.

I helped Chris sit up. He was very emotional, and physically felt very cold, despite his sweating. Andrew and I both knew we were looking at a changed man. Physically there was no obvious alteration, but soulfully he had moved more into who he really is. On that night we could see Chris more brightly than before. And time showed us even more.

Recounting some of the experience to us, he told me how he had felt his eyes opening but couldn't stop them. He then said, "I looked at you, Mel, but you looked different. I knew it was you, even though you looked different. And you flickered in and out like an old film. I tried to close my eyes then I saw the other lady, on the other side of the table. She was looking at me just like you were. She had long dark wavy hair, but she was like you. She smiles like you do, too."

Chris was one of the first of many to use that phrase; "I looked at you, but you looked different. I knew it was you, even though you looked different…" I still hear it often from clients.

Chris gave me a gift of lesson, perhaps because I was so at ease with this friend that I adore, I was able to turn his session into my classroom. And so very much came out of this session.

For me it was confirmation that this healing process had indeed changed and developed even more. I was seeing it client by client, and yet, as it is with your own children, you aren't able to see the bigger picture until someone else points out how much your child has grown or changed since they last saw them.

Immersed as I was in the action, an objective, or even a blanket overview was near impossible. The combination of Chris's experience, Andrew's perspective and hence ability to offer this newer objective view of the growth and change, as well as my own experience as the vehicle, culminated in a personal shift for me, Melissa, and a dramatic shift in frequencies and in healing.

I knew it was working, of this I had no doubts. People were walking in with any number of ailments and thirty minutes later leaving without them. However, a month or two before working with Chris I had begun to question just how effective an instrument I was in applying this process of healing. How efficient or effective was I in session? Working on children is what originally made me address this question, this doubt. One little girl with epilepsy was the trigger and a new class of lesson.

She was only nine, and had multiple absence or petit mal seizures (brief episodes of staring), per day, as well as the very occasional grand mal seizure. Both parents came in with her, and the session started.

Children simply fly during session. They take off rapidly and their registers and response at this end, in session, can be huge. This little girl was like that.

From the outset her sweet little face started to shift dramatically from a frown, to a huge smile, to a seriously concerned expression, and many others in a series of extreme expressions. Her arms started to occasionally fling out sideways. Soon after her legs joined the party and started to intermittently twitch.

Bear in mind I love doing this, and especially so with kids, so I was really enjoying this session and I turned to smile encouragingly at her parents. The concern on their face was plain. Clearly they thought she was in seizure, although their querying looks suggested it was unlike any other they had witnessed. I tried to reassure them with small comforting gestures, indicating all was normal, but my mind was racing.

This little girl was deep in session. And this session was important for her. More than most parents I truly can empathise with the distress of watching your child struggle or suffer, as I live it daily. I needed to find a way of continuing this session, before the parent's distress interrupted it.

I dropped my hands away, in the hope of reducing the flow, but at this stage the little girl was charged, the frequency flowing rich and potent about her and moving my hands away had no affect in reducing her physical response. I needed to alter the flow of the frequencies. I had danced around this for a few months, but now it was crunch time.

I lifted my hands again, just feeling her body's response under my hands, and ***deliberately reduced the flow of the frequency*** through myself. Almost like I was smoothing it out, I moved about her, watching as her gross motor registers, arms and legs, and head movement ceased almost instantaneously. Her eyes, however, continued to oscillate beneath the eyelids, even more rapidly, but as evenly and as rhythmically as before.

Her parents sighed audibly. And I took on their distressed internal questioning, as I asked myself if I had done the session an injustice. I was blown away that I was able to instrumentally alter the flow, which was pretty cool actually. But had this alteration diminished the ultimate exposure, and hence this little girl's session?

The session ended, and instantly I put Dad in front of her. The first thing kids need after a session is a huge cuddle with someone that they love. (*Note to Healers, put that in your notes. It's important.*) After her hug, she started to recount what she had experienced. Who she had seen, a beautiful lady, a talking giraffe, swans you could ride on, and what they had said to her. And how she had wished she didn't have to come back.

Her session had not been disrupted. Her experience was no less, and she had felt no conscious change physically, except that somewhere along the way she felt "like I could relax more". I had to consider that to simplify the physical response of the client, to reduce that which is consciously distracting at my end of it, could enhance the experience for the client.

The human being, as any living creature or organism, is in a constant state of evolution. Try as we have throughout history, we cannot hope to win the battle against evolution. And we have tried, in so many arenas; religion, politics, economically, environmentally. It takes little imagination, and a whole lot of courage, when one looks upon our history, to see the dogmatism running rife. Yet also in that is history, one thing is clear; any attempts to stifle or to stagnate evolution, are futile.

Quantum frequencies show themselves to be readily present, and to cause such extraordinary healing ability, and because it's within the comfort zone, we assume that that is all there is. We waved our hands about, things started to happen, and …that's it? No. That's not "it" at all. That is ego. Our conscious mindset, even our desire for money, will only get run over if it stands in the way of an evolution like this.

Energy healing is a gift we've known for sometime. Anyone wise would expect energy healing to be enhanced, and allow for it to evolve as it inevitably would. These newly present frequencies, quantum based, are evidence of that process of evolution. The session, with this epileptic child, demonstrated to me the need, the requirement, for me to look for that enhancement, for that evolved "next step"!

Only weeks before this session, as I had been in session with another client, I had received one of the two frequent messages I tend to receive: that there was "more to follow".

Of course there would be *more to follow*!

As I had, in my quest to understand this more, been speaking to various healers and authors, I had come across a number that had turned "healing" into a multi million dollar business. Unfortunately for them, they had caused for themselves stagnation in both their healing ability, and in their business, as they had cornered themselves into marketing a stagnant product. I had already in my privileged objective position been witness to this. And in witnessing this I decided that I would *always* do client sessions personally, as I knew this where I would be guided and I would learn.

I have also come across some amazing mentors, (you'll see a number of them quoted throughout this volume) who despite their marketable assets have kept true to their healing modality in lieu of "selling out" in order to stay true to their teaching, thankfully.

We, the team at **melissa hocking healing**, and with Quantum BioEnergetics International, while continuing to teach, also continue to allow for the enhancement and the evolution. The facilitators that have trained with us are always welcome to come back and update their notes, and to enhance and hone their application, as we do not pretend at any stage that this is complete. We're also always open to learning. ***Ancora Imparo***. We just aren't obnoxious enough to believe we know it all!

To your benefit, healing facilitator, for as mind blowing and beautiful as it is, that you have found this, there will be *more to follow*.

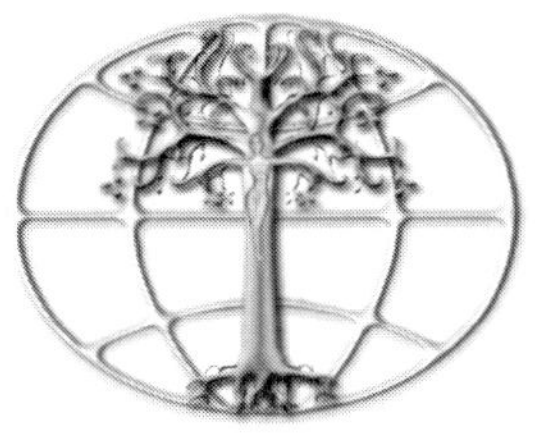

The "How"

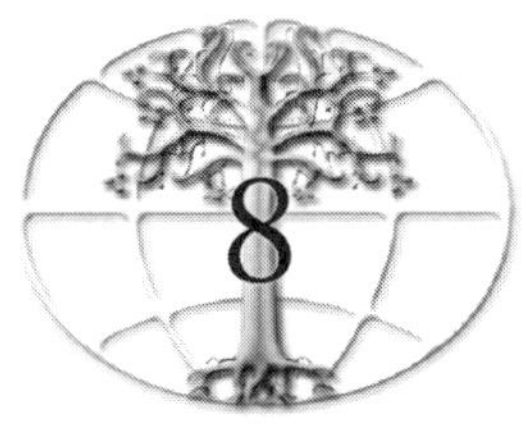

"There are no such things as miracles, only unknown laws."
St Augustine

The "How"

H*ow is the living body responding like this?*

It's a given that I have to offer some explanation of what is going on within the human body, for it to heal of ailments considered incurable by any other means. People come in the door of my healing rooms with terminal illness, chronic disease, permanent disabilities and walk out, now knowing that these issues are no longer "terminal", "chronic" or "permanent". What is occurring in the rooms of facilitators utilizing this form of healing?

Facts. Scientific, measurable, linear evidence. That's what I wanted. It should be enough, shouldn't it, that the results are amazing and speak for themselves? But its not. The very nature of being human is that the conscious mind requires that external input, extrinsically sourced confirmation, before launching in new uncharted realms. Deepak Chopra says of this, "*Unless we have scientific validations for healing methods they will always be put into the category of superstition.*" In order for this to be available to all who may need it, to reach a broader population than the "believers", we had to find more readily acceptable validation.

Earlier I mentioned that our history, and learning henceforth, in Western medicine placed us in such a position that we would believe what was happening, or healing us, was from an external influence applied to a body causing a reaction or response. Appropriately at the time, we would readily place responsibility for our health and well being extrinsically.

It's no accident that a common recognition addressing cell and DNA vibrations is occurring. Within the living cell is a molecule consisting of the entire genetic coding of an individual which we refer to as DNA. When we think of DNA we tend to visualize a helix, neat and orderly, twisting uniformly upon itself, for those are the images fed to us. From the outset of our knowledge of human DNA, we were shown a double helix; two strands of DNA. In reality its appearance is anything but orderly. Already, even in our perception of only two strands, when viewed you see an incredibly complex vibrating matrix.

More and more so, that which I perceived to be a recognition dawning from within the body has begun to be proven to be true.

Enormous revelations are dawning upon us. Modern research has started to not only show evidence of string theory (bloody exciting in itself), giving weight to quantum physics and the possibility of measurement thereof, but also we now have evidence of the actual vibration of the recognized helix itself, leading us to recognize that the changes that are occurring in the human body, the healings, are evidently, at the very core and essence of us; from within at a cellular level. And not through any addition or alteration, or external application on the facilitators part, but instead, through *memory* within the cell itself! From within!

Now with scientific advances, just as we have recently visually recognized a planet outside our own solar system, scientists are also starting to recognize the pattern of DNA to extend far beyond the double helix originally seen. Various sources including ancient scripture, channelled writing, and even some brave souls in the scientific community are now willing to address the possibility, even the likelihood, of 12 layers of human DNA. 12. Yes, 12.

For some time I was lead to believe that what was occurring when a body was exposed to these frequencies was not just a triggering of DNA, or of what was referred to as dormant DNA junk, but instead, an alteration. Actually what they were suggesting to me was a *creation* of the DNA. My gut feeling was "no". That answer felt incomplete. Especially as those trying to convince me, considered the question answered, and that we needed to seek no more. Fortunately, other sources were venturing to a point suggesting that we were, in facilitation, re-establishing DNA to its original inter-dimensional 12 layer matrix, instead of the double helix (2 strands) that we are all familiar with. More of a *recreation.* This opens a can of worms, doesn't it?

I know this can of worms all too well, as I have spent a great amount of time, energy and research committed to understanding and answering it for myself. One thing I knew for sure was that the information that I did have was incomplete. I just wasn't satisfied with the "I don't knows" that were being handed to me when I queried it.

Fortunately, recent studies are soaring on the wings of absolutely astonishing evidence. String theory, newly "suspected" strands of DNA, and cellular regeneration, are all speaking up through science more loudly and clearly than ever. Biology itself is advancing at a rate unparalleled. You scientists out there must be beside yourselves with excitement!

Several groups across the planet, through their research, have recently come to evidence of the DNA helix actually vibrating under certain frequencies leading to the progressive conclusion that healing can and is occurring from the cell itself.

One of the most intriguing and yet, not so surprising cases, is through personal interactions with dolphins, in a program for dolphin assisted therapy. Dr Michael Hyson and a team of Cetacean researchers based at the Sirius Institute in Hawaii have recently published a report (*DNA: Pirates of the Sacred Spiral*) that examines DNA's coiled design, vibrating action, and electromagnetic functions during bioacoustic interactions between dolphins and humans. Their ongoing study shows that these marine mammals receive and transmit sound signals capable of effecting the genetic double helix of the human, and using natural biotechnology, dolphins may heal humans immersed in the water near them sonogenetically. This report addresses DNA's coiled design, vibrating action and electro genetic functions during bioacoustic interactions between dolphins and humans.

Earlier, we discussed balance, and that the healer's role is not to heal, but to create balance so that the body, that community of cells, becomes an environment in which it can *heal itself.* What this particular report is able to give evidence to is more the resonance occurring between two individuals, where the dolphin is the facilitator, creating a balanced environment, using sonar to cause the DNA helix (that is visible) to vibrate. From this a deeper and even more extraordinary event occurs; at a cellular level, the body is able to repair itself.

Cells; Cells are the very base make up of human, and other living, biology. We've all had some experience at viewing cells even if your only recollection was a crude experiment in high school science from some badly dismembered plant.

So we're all pretty familiar with the basic make up, biologically of the cell; membrane, atoms, molecules, etc. And that is what we know, what we are comfortable in recognizing, of a biological cell as the human in duality.

Imagine a single cell. Within that cell, in that single cell, is the entire make up of who you are. Everything that you would do, you would be, and that you have, is housed within the vibration of that single cell. For contained in that cell is you; the real you, the absolute you. For that cell is perfect. That cell *is* ***You.***

Gregg Braden writes "*The hate, disease and suffering in our world, as well as the love, healing and miracles are manifestations of our inner selves, longing to be heard, acknowledged and answered.*" Perhaps more importantly, in that cell the memory of whom you are, the real you, the *spirit* that is you, resides. Kryon refers to "*the angel that you are*" within that cell.

The good stuff; each living cell has a naturally occurring vibration that relates to its level of mass, form and energy, and hence to the environment in which it is vibrating. The helix itself, when viewed is vibrating; a vibration, an energy, a *frequency*. Remember frequency is based on light and information, not "energy" per se, and so it makes sense that each individual cell has a naturally occurring vibration.

This concept isn't new, either. In cancer studies particularly, they are all over the possibility of altering the cell's reception to the changes that trigger cancerous growth and to the possibility of self recovery, of self healing. Studies and treatment at this stage are leaning toward electromagnetic interference, EM frequencies. Nutritional studies are showing a number of direct effects as well; certain aspartame products directly effecting the cell membrane, or trans-fatty acids altering cell function entirely almost immediately after assimilation, and many more cellular responses attributed to our nutritional intake alone.

So if those cells are "perfect", Melissa, why do I still have cellulite? Yeah, I hear you.

As yet, we aren't yet operating at our maximum. There are parts of those "gaps" in the matrix that are yet to be activated. To explain.....

Let's take, for example, a Formula 1 racing car (the human body). A beautiful thing (yes, I am a fan, both of Formula 1, and the human body). This is the precision built, absolute elite racing car. Its engine is highly and finely tuned, managed to perfection, and capable of achieving speeds and performance above any other racing vehicle in existence. The body of this car is designed and built to exacting standards; correct down force, weight distributions, balance. This is the ***premiere racing vehicle*** on this planet. However currently, there is a disabling element occurring in this vehicle; the gearbox isn't able to complete its "go between". The exquisite and extraordinary engine is unable to propel the vehicle, because it is unable to communicate *adequately*, or *accurately*, with the other appropriate parts of the car. Until the avenues of communication are triggered, this divine vehicle cannot know the depth of its potential. On its own the engine is incredible to behold, in its design. A disembodied engine is still a beautiful thing, but immovable nonetheless. Yet when the gearbox (DNA) is triggered appropriately, and can then communicate with all elements that make up this vehicle, it can become all it should be.

This very matrix, DNA, put in the right environment, under certain frequencies, can reactivate and re-establish communication with the cellular database. Latest findings suspect that the DNA isn't causing this, it is enabling it.

Scientists in the past couple decades have made huge advances in working with DNA. The discovery of the effect of certain enzymes affecting, and actually severing the DNA, moved us into the possibility of manipulating DNA, and even the synthetic reproduction of DNA. Nowadays, genetic modification has been applied to plant life, animal, and now, as we are all aware, they are trying to address the possibility of modifying the human genome.

Recent papers have shown that collectively, scientists are just in the infancy of looking at the effect of vibration, on DNA and ultimately its effect on the genome. These incredible doctors and scientists are coming together globally looking at possibilities for healing and recovery. Okay, healing and recovery, amongst other uses for genetic manipulation. Let us stick to the topic of healing.

When a client is in a quantum bioenergetic session, you, as the facilitator, immerse the client's body within these incredible quantum based frequencies. As the instrument or vehicle you create an environment of balance, an environment in which the body can select to heal itself. What seems to be occurring is a *whole body entrainment*, as each cell is accessed via the extraordinary communication, the interpreter known as human DNA.

Each cell, housing absolute memory of you, will select an appropriate healing for you. Certainly at a physical level, but also far deeper and more intrinsically, there too is balance, awakening, healing. I mentioned it before; a "whole body entrainment".

Gregg Braden explains it: "*A coded message discovered deep within the DNA of each living cell provides concrete evidence that we are related not only to one another, but to all life, in the most intimate way.*"

As complex as this sounds, and as heavy as it may be to read, it is yours. This form of healing seems to actually change the vibration that your body is operating at, raising it, allowing for the communication of the DNA matrix with the cellular body and hence the entire body. From here it initiates not only permission to heal, but the power to heal, using information that has always been there, but until now we had been unable to access.

And it's yours; to heal yourself, to heal others, to assist

your veggie garden, or your incontinent Labrador, if you so choose. Because what is also yours, always, is choice. You can choose to use this or not. You can choose to utterly ignore it. You can choose how you use it. For even if you own nothing else, already you own this incredible ability to heal.

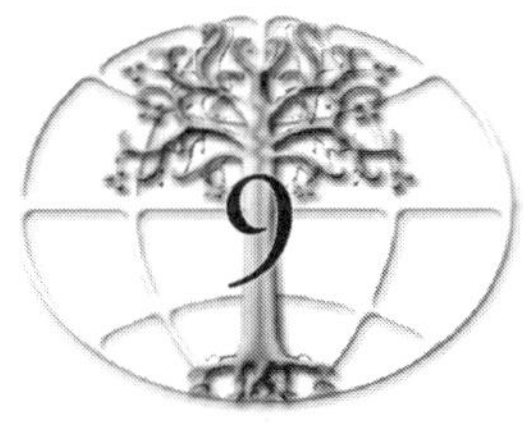

"Real mysteries lie in what is seen, not unseen."
Spanish proverb

Discovering the incredible gift...within You

F*inally* we get to it! This is the single moment for which I do this: the reason that I write for you now, or teach the courses that I do in healing, lecture to any number of groups, or continue to do private client sessions.

The moment when *you* get it. When *you* feel this in *your* hands, palpable and present; of you, within you, about you. It is why I do what I do, to pass this amazing gift on. I love this!

Before we get in to the nitty-gritty of just where and how to "find" this gift, I think you should know, you've already found it. You already have it. I offer you no miracles here, because *you are* the miracle. This is your gift, of you, within you, for you to use or not. No amount of summoning or manifesting or meditating or manipulating can bring this on, or make it disappear. From the moment you recognize these frequencies within you they will only become more palpable, stronger, whether you use them regularly or not. You may never use them or investigate them at all for twelve years, then one day say to yourself, "*I wonder if they're still there...*" and, bang, you'll feel them stronger and more present than ever.

And so, the first introduction to these frequencies, is exactly that; a recognition, an introduction to a gift already within. Now I understand that identifying something you've never found before, could sound a little difficult. You'll find that these frequencies are far simpler than you imagine. My advice to you; *keep* it simple.

You can imagine how much I have toiled with the concept of describing this to you. When each body is so unique, surely, for each person, this will feel slightly different. How can I describe a feeling you've never felt before?

Initially I tend to introduce this process through your hands. Whenever I speak to groups or individuals about this, as people approach and ask questions about it, I'll say "Would you like to feel it?" and because it's easiest, and least physically intrusive, I simply trigger the frequencies about their hands. (The great bonus in this for me is I get a real sensation of the individual I'm working with, even in a crowded and chaotic public environment.)

In the healing facilitation courses we teach, in one room of fifty people, everyone feels and describes these frequencies differently. One gentleman will have something similar to a bubble effect, a consistent pressure all about his hand, while another woman feels like a bar protrudes through the palm of her hand (not painfully, just present). Occasionally, although not often, someone feels nothing from their own hands and that is normal too.

However, the beauty of these frequencies is they have some very distinct and (fortunately) obvious signals that it is present and that we are quite clearly interacting with it. Of course you will feel it, as will the people you work with when facilitating this process, but an added bonus is that you can actually watch these frequencies at work.

A shift occurred, a personal shift just for you, when you made the decision to seek this information out. Already your connection with these frequencies, with this healing ability, has been growing, initiating and developing, as you have been reading. Your next step certainly, is to physically feel it palpably in yourself. Yet, this step requires you to prepare for it.

Belief. Not faith. This is not faith healing. This isn't about hope, it's about knowledge.

In Star Wars, Luke Skywalker is being trained by Yoda, Jedi master, and when Yoda demonstrates the power of "the force", Luke gasps, awestruck, "I don't believe it!"

And Yoda replies, "*That* is why you fail."

If you do not believe in the source, your ability to transfer these frequencies is altered, even hindered. They will not flow. A lack of belief never stands alone, particularly a lack of belief in the source; ultimately it is a lack of belief in you.

In such moments ego takes the opportunity to step in, fear finds an entry point, and your self esteem, and your ability as a healing facilitator, take a beating. Sadly, I've seen it many times in healing practitioners during workshops and courses. It starts as disbelief in essence, then that competitive one-upmanship kicks in, that leads to jealousy, resentment, ridiculous superficial emotional crap, really. And the ability to initiate healing dissipates. Through their bolstering and self proclamation they try to compensate, but remember some of us can actually see these frequencies, or the lack thereof. Pretence gets you nowhere in this.

All great men have known times of discord when fear gained entry upon their mind.

Initiating through the hands

As I mentioned, a great introductory environment for this is in the hands, and that is, even in this book, where we'll begin.

The hands, like the feet, contain one of the largest concentrations of energy response points in the human biology, mirroring that very biology and the human energy systems. This is not a new concept. Reflexologists, among other practitioners, will tell you that the sole of the foot represents all functional, energetic systems in the physiological process. The hands housing a number of meridian exit points of the human anatomy, among various other energy "exchange" ports, are a rich source of light transferral (information). Viewing the human anatomy as the whole resonant instrument, the hands (and feet) are primary investigatory tools, with their concentrated collective of frequency feedback, however they are not isolated in their function. Always remember the whole of our being exists as an interconnecting collection of systems.

This is one of the easiest places to start to teach. We're so conscious of using our hands to do the simplest of tasks; so used to physical sensation within them, that it is an obvious place to start. (That being said, the use of your hands in the application of this healing process is not *essential* at all.)

When I'm activating these frequencies about a person's hand I ask them to place their hand, relaxed, in front of them. If you've been involved in other healing techniques particularly, a relaxed position for the hand can be hard to do. You want your hand in a simple, anatomical position. The best way to do this is to drop your hands to your sides, and just kind of shake your arms out as you would if you had tension in your shoulders. Then, without looking at your hand, or altering the position your hand is in, bend at the elbow and raise your hand up in front of you so that your forearm is at ninety degrees to your upper arm. Now, without altering it at all, look at your hand. You found it.

The position that the hand is in is known as a "normal anatomic position" (*See Diagram I in Appendix 1*). Try this process again now and have a look at the position your hand is in. This is a controlled position; don't just let your hand flop. There should be no muscular tension in the hand at all; a slight bend in all the finger joints so that an even curve occurs through the fingers, and the fingers are apart from one another. The wrist tilts back slightly. One of the telltale signs that you have it is if it's comfortable. (The human body was designed for comfort, you know.)

When your hand is in this position you'll notice that it is an "open" position. That is key in the transference of these frequencies. This open position allows for flow, and you'll find, overlays all aspects of this form of healing.

What I then do, when activating somebody's hand, is place my hands on either side of theirs, palms facing toward each other so that my hands are about a foot or so apart. And this incredible energy flows…

William A. Tiller, PhD, wrote, "*One way of accelerating the desired transformation in individuals and societies is via human energy-field interactions*".

When I do demonstrate this to a client, while the physical sensation is palpable and quite obvious, visually there is a change in the hands too. Most commonly, quite a visible mottled effect occurs. Patchy colouring on the palm and fingers, and sometimes a little puffing up of the flesh will happen. None of this is painful, and it dissipates as soon as I desist. For some whenever they trigger the frequencies through their hands this will occur. In my own hands still, I experience this. It seems another gentle confirmation that yes, this is flowing, and yes, it is working.

Gregg Braden in his book *Walking Between the Worlds*, defines this interactive process as an *entrainment*; an alignment of forces, or fields of energy, to allow maximum transfer of information or communication. He goes on to refer to the synchronization of two or more elements, to a common and usually higher vibration, when interacting together.

To me it's clear that this is exactly what occurs when one individual introduces these frequencies to another. Almost instantaneously both are able to vibrate with these incredible frequencies, at the same level.

When I initiate this for someone, I simply find it, gently feeling the play of energy between my own hands, interacting in and around the person's hand. Almost instantly you get a response from the other person's body, the sensation flowing from and through them becomes distinct and I am able to enhance their flow. I then effectively "stretch" the energy by moving my own hands further away from the person's, and hence, as is the nature of these quantum based frequencies, intensify the flow of them.

These frequencies are palpable, the sensation quite physical, and I'm yet to have someone not experience this unmistakable sensation in one way or another. People report it in various ways; some have heat, some cold, there can be pulling or pushing, a breezy sensation, a pressure, tingling, buzzing, and throbbing. None is right or wrong, for as I said, each individual in their physical individuality, is bound to experience it in their own way.

What's occurring at a physical level for the human, as the body recognizes these frequencies, is where we are still working to prove scientifically. As we've mentioned earlier, there are a variety of theories as to what is actually occurring at a DNA level, when a body is exposed to these frequencies during a healing session. However this situation, this reintroduction between an individual body and these frequencies, seems to bring about a unique and somewhat separate response. There is a point of recognition, far more tangible consciously for the person experiencing it.

This, the sensation you feel in your hands, is where you have to consider that even though we're still in the process of proving it scientifically, the memory of this comes from within. The theories of an extrinsic element, alien, spiritual or otherwise, beyond our interaction or control, insult the real source. In this moment, as never before, you start to see the enormous potential of a single human being. Just from this initial exposure and awakening, the shift is immense and very personal for each person; a momentary point in Your evolution.

But as I am not in the room right now to initiate this for you, so let's get on with the business of helping you to find it.

Feel your hands.

Shake out your shoulders, but this time, leave your hands in that relaxed anatomical position at your sides.

Now what I want you to do is to remember when you made the decision to read this book. Where were you? What were you doing? What was going on in your head? Perhaps consciously you were thinking it might be an interesting read, or someone had recommended it and somewhere deeper, somewhere within perhaps you knew, or at least hoped, that maybe, just maybe, there was something special in this book that could help you. Do you remember that need to heal, that desire to help others, perhaps a need to help someone special? Do you want to heal yourself? Do you want to help others? Think back and remember. Remember the moment you picked up the book and opened the page to read. Can you see it in your mind?

Do you intend to recognize this feeling, these frequencies, in your hands? If the answer is "yes", then say it out loud. Remember conscious intent plays no small role here. Recognizing the ability for humans to heal such as this, through immersion within quantum based frequency, in itself brings about intent, and hence activation from within you.

Now, feel your hands next to your body. Leaving them

where they are, keeping your arms relaxed and straight, tilt your wrist backwards, away from the body so that the palm of your hand faces the floor. Your hand remains in a relaxed position. Try not to extend your fingers, or stiffen your hand. This position is the extreme version of an open position, and for a reason. You're about to feel that reason…

Gently take a deep breath and as you breathe out you will feel your neck, and shoulders relax. Without changing your arm, wrist or hand's position lift your shoulders up, shrug upward, hold them there for a moment, and then drop them. Just drop them, don't control the movement. Try it again, this time focus on the feeling in your hands and lift your shoulders, then drop them.

Can you feel the weight drop through your hand? If not, try it again. Remain relaxed, take a breath, relax your upper body again, then raise your shoulders…and drop.

This doesn't dissipate either. Do it again and again and you'll find the sensation is no less. I find I play with this gift, all the time. When I go for a run, I have a track that winds for a few kilometres through a reserve that is an exquisite bush area. As I run beneath the ancient gum trees with each step it's like ten-kilogram weights drop from each of my hands.

Discovering it

Let's find it in you.

Once more, I ask you to drop the "energy" through your hands, but this time focus on the sensation as it lands in your hands. Lift your shoulders…

During this exercise, the sensation lands in the palm of your hand, focused mainly in the area around the top of the palm, opposite the first knuckle of the middle finger.

For the more auditory learners, this is the palmer side of the hand, at the proximal IP joint of the middle finger. For those that are visual see A*ppendix 1, diagram II* for a visual map.

This point is known as through traditional Chinese medicine as the "pericardium 8", as it is the eighth point on the pericardium meridian channel. Earlier I mentioned the hands' receptive role as several meridians exit the human energy anatomy through them. Not by accident you will notice that as you drop the frequencies through your hands, the concentrated point of sensation is directly at this point: the pericardium 8.

Throughout any of the exercises I have for you in here, unless it's suggested otherwise, watch what you are doing. Keep your eyes on the action. Don't close your eyes as you try to focus on the feeling, or in order to concentrate better. I mentioned before that a significant percentage of these frequencies come through my eyes, at any time, or even most of it if I choose. You don't need to look at your hands; you can look away, *but don't close your eyes.*

After dropping the frequencies into your hands, bring your hands up in front of you, in their relaxed, open, anatomical position. Now select your favourite hand, (without getting too technical) and let's get started. Look at your hand…

Imagine that a pencil, just a normal sized wooden pencil, is *painlessly* sticking through that pericardium 8 point in your palm, protruding on either side of the hand. (It would have suited me better to use a scarf through your hand, rather than a pencil, but it wouldn't have been so easy to describe how to grasp it) With the other hand, you're going to effectively pull that pencil through your hand. So slowly bring your open hand toward the "pencil", your palm approaching the end of it, and using all five digits (fingers and thumb) uniformly bring the tips of the fingers together around the imaginary pencil. The tips of your fingers should only be one or two inches away from the palm of your other hand when you bring them together. Remember there is a pencil there, so the tips of your fingers won't be touching one another as you slowly draw your hand back, pulling the pencil through your hand. Try it again, going back to that same point. *See Diagram III in Appendix 1.*

Try to keep your pace uniform too as you're drawing your hand back, so you get maximum sensation. When doing this for the first time, it can take two or three attempts before you get a really good feel for it. Those primary sensations will start on the second or third attempt, (the breeze, or a pull, perhaps a buzz) and will become exponentially more pronounced with each try. Once you've got it, you've got it.

Slowly draw your hand back thirty to fifty centimetres perpendicular to the palm housing the PC8 point, and you'll notice that the pencil actually has no end. It keeps coming.

Now reverse each hand's role, and try it from your other hand. Play with it! The frequencies are based in quantum physics, and get *stronger with distance.* As you familiarize yourself with the sensation, *feel* how the frequencies draw through, *where* they are drawing from.

Now that you are activated, now that you are a vehicle, a conduit for the transference of these frequencies of immense light and information, we can move on to exactly what we have initiated… Let's play.

An exercise to enhance…

The exercises I'm going to give you so that you can recognize and enhance your knowledge of your gift are kind of graduated through developmental grades. So if you've lost the sensation, or aren't quite getting it for some reason, go back to the previous exercise, and regain that familiarity before you try again.

Back to base, getting ready to play again, do the old, shakeout your shoulders, tilt your wrists back, lift your shoulders and drop…Feel it.

Drop your wrists, so that your hands are by your sides,

and bending at the elbow, bring your hands up in front of you in their relaxed anatomical position.

You are familiar now with the concentrated point on the palm of your hand, level with the knuckle of the middle finger, pericardium 8, where the frequencies most obviously flow. Bring your hands together, one palm facing up, one facing down, palm over palm, about two inches or so apart. Looking at you hands, try to line up the two concentrated points one over the other.

Imagine now that between the two points is a chunk of Playdough, only a few square centimetres of it, and you're going to slowly roll that chunk into a ball. Keep your lower hand stationary, and using your upper hand, start to *slowly* form that ball of playdough between those two concentrated points.

The movement is more in the tilting of your wrist than in making huge circles around the lower hand. Note speed is not your ally at this stage. Keep it slow and feel for it. Distinctly you will feel the ball in your hand! Cool, isn't it?

Are your eyes open? I hope so, otherwise you are more of a freak of nature than I am, if you're reading this with your eyes closed! Don't shut your eyes.

Snowballing…

Once you can clearly feel the little ball, add a bigger chunk of playdough. Take a good look at the palm of your hand, and mentally place upon it a circular coaster. Yes, like the ones you put your drink on. This time your palms are more like three or four inches apart, one palm over the other. Using your top hand, move the concentrated point around the edge of your coaster, and roll that ball of play dough. *Appendix 1, diagram IV.*

Moving about a larger "ball", you want to tilt the palm of your upper hand as it moves around the perimeter so that the connection of the energy is always to the centre of the palm of your lower hand. Imagine a beam going from the concentration point of your upper hand to the centre of the palm of your lower hand, and your upper hand will roll about the ball of play dough. *Appendix 1, diagram V.*

What you don't want is to be drawing a flat circle around and around over the top of your other hand. Try both techniques, and you'll understand. The difference is distinct.

The motion isn't the goal. You want to *feel* this… enhance it. Feel it. This education is experiential, sourced from within.

What exactly will you feel?

The very palpable nature of these frequencies can be interpreted via any number of sensations by your own body, and will be. Each person experiences the flow of these frequencies, feeling it physically through their body differently. Each body is ultimately constructed uniquely, so slightly differing sensations aren't that much of a surprise.

These frequencies may talk through your body through any or even all of these sensations:

- Cool breeze
- Buzzing
- Pressure
- Temperature
- Tingling
- Many tiny droplets raining upon your hands,
- A fog or uniform pressure
- Pulling
- Pushing
- A viscous, fluid motion
- An elastic stretch
- Many more interpretations

There are one or two sensations that are commonly experienced during your introduction to these frequencies. Not everyone feels them, but most will. As you develop your recognition and your knowledge of working with these frequencies, many more auspices and nuances will come in, differing sensations, primarily, however, these frequencies will be present. Their consistency aids us in introducing this to people, and allowing them to recognize them at their own pace. So what's first?

A cool breeze, about, around or through (any of these or all of them) the hand. No it's not the air conditioning. And no it's not because you're waving your hands about. You were meant to be doing this slowly, remember? Or have you been reading with your eyes closed again?

Commonly, and usually just as the person you're introducing to the frequencies is picking their jaw up off the floor, a new sensation registers on top of the breeze: a buzzing. It's a strange term "buzzing", but when you feel it you'll understand. There really is no other way to describe this sensation.

Other sensations come in on top again, and you will feel a pulling or a pushing, a tingling or the buzzing moves up your arms, palpably. Quite incredible that the frequencies are felt so readily and palpably, isn't it?

I seriously consider the fact that these frequencies introduced themselves in this process of healing that crude physical matter we walk about in, the human biology, so that we, the human, would invite this change and embrace it. And, of course, we *are* embracing it.

If you had doubts, and you may, as to whether these frequencies really existed or not, you can just check yourself again. And there they are. This gift is yours. If you're anything like I was, you'll be stopped at the traffic lights and rolling the ball between your hands without even thinking.

Used or not, these frequencies get stronger and more

palpable with time. Of course used, the sensation and innate knowledge of these frequencies causes them to develop more quickly, but regardless this is your gift. The only person that can take it from you is you.

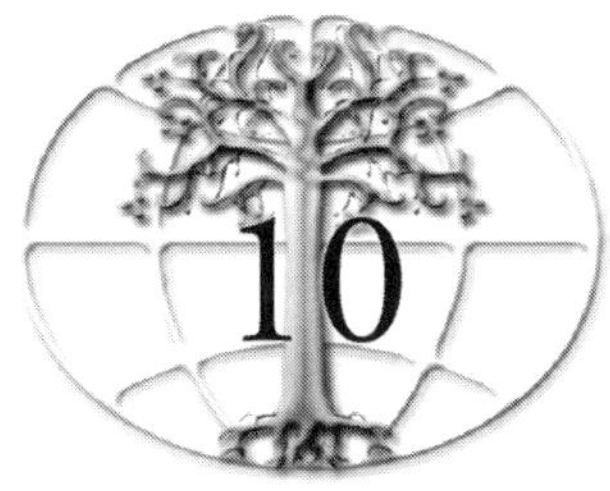

"No understanding of evolution is adequate that does not have at its core that we are on a journey to authentic power, and that authentic empowerment is the goal of our evolutionary process and the purpose of our being."
Gary Zukav

The Road Ahead

Every child is born into a different family. Every child is raised in a different and ever-changing house.

I was raised within the Christian religion, Catholic to be precise. I went to Catholic church, Catholic schools, the whole bit. Somehow along the way, I hadn't been baptized. A blessing in disguise for me as in order to get into the catholic school my parents wanted me to attend, I had to be. This is where I started my search into religions, theology and ultimately, essentially spirituality. I spent a lot of time with our local priest, a young gentleman who was not averse to my questions and curiosity. In fact, when I suggested what I wanted to do, the pastor, Father Luff loved the idea and couldn't wait to put it into action.

A beautiful river called the Tambo River surrounded the property we lived on, and I had requested a full immersion baptism, in it. When asked who I would choose for godparents, my choice was easy: my adopted grandmother, Aunty Ze, the most beautiful woman in the world. Although I was concerned about burdening this already enormously generous lady with my spiritual guidance as well.

Then I found a loophole in the doctrine. I decided instead that I would be baptized as an adult (I was eleven) so that I could be my own godparent and therefore direct my own spiritual guidance. Word got around about this event, and on the day I walked down the gentle sandy bank to the river's edge, hundreds stood upon the river bank to bear witness.

Father Luff was obviously enjoying the attendance, for I nearly drowned as he slowly and dramatically intoned prayer while I was immersed. My lasting conscious memory of the whole event is the sensation of exploding lungs desperate for oxygen. (Sadly, Father Luff was later expelled from the church when he fell in love with a wonderful woman. He now has two beautiful children and a wonderful life. But it was another moment in time that brought far more questions than answers about the religion I was to behold.)

And so I entered the intended Catholic secondary school. A fabulous school, rich in opportunity and education, and very pious religion. I attended mass three times a week (more if it was around Easter or Lent), assembly twice a week and chapel once a week where I was to repent in earnest solitude.

My ears constantly rang with "You are a sinner!" "You must confess" "Repent, Melissa, repent", and I was told that God held me in judgment, I would be judged, I would be punished for my sins and that Satan, fire, brimstone, and damnation were inevitably upon me. (Can you imagine an Indigo in this environment? Cosmic humour at it's best!) I was the penultimate sinner, particularly in my teenage years.

I can still recall one of the brothers that taught at the school I attended, when I had been quizzing him during biblical studies, wheeling about on me and spitting,

"Melissa! Do your feet feel warm?"

"No. Why?"

"They should! For surely the very molten beds of Hell itself are beneath your feet!"

So by the time I was eighteen I was pretty much an atheist.

But always, I knew there was more.

Thankfully the Catholic Church I have privilege to see, and occasionally speak at these days, is so much more evolved than the church I grew up in.

Around fourteen or fifteen I had started soaking up books on the Dead Sea scrolls, by various theologians, some quite "out there", which lead into the study of various religions. It became a quiet joke between my father and I. We would be sitting on the step of the veranda, in silence, resting side by side, and he would turn to me with a cheeky smirk and say "So what is it this week? Are you a Scientologist? A Buddhist? Jehovah's?" Such a question was of course my cue to talk about what I had discovered, since we last sat together on that veranda step.

Dad's theory on why I was like this went back to when I was only four or five. Mum and Dad went away for a few days, and I stayed with friends of theirs. It turned out they were devotes of Hare Krishna. I came home with new clothes in orange and yellow and pink, telling Mum and Dad that "Christians were hypocrites." Ah, the simple joys of childhood.

I left home at eighteen, entering university and the workforce all at once. And the spiritual journey intensified. Pentecostal churches where every man and his dog seemed to have the ability to speak in tongues. Apocalyptic churches recruiting for mass annihilation at the turn of the millennium.

I did delve into Scientology, Hinduism, and Mormon. I even joined Amway for a while, but it was too intense (just kidding! I'm still in Amway; great products).

I kept reaching out and hungrily so, for I knew there was more and I knew it would come to me. The human child within me just wanted to be accepted, in the hope of perhaps being loved. The spirit that is me knew better.

Just as the spirit that is you, knows better.

The path that is yours to travel is simple. But it is not easy.

For each of us is on this planet with purpose. Each individual that comes into your life is there with purpose, so that you can grow, and learn, and reach out a little further. I know it hasn't been easy for you. Some of you have suffered heinous abuse, or appalling traumas, or incredible loneliness, and much more. While I do not endorse the method by which you were forced to attain it, I do know that within you, born from those hideous experiences, is strength unbeknownst to most people. It is a strength that has lent you the courage to seek "something" more; a strength that has lead you here, now.

We cannot let the blinders of our upbringing, the history of this single life thwart us from the journey ahead. For our role is far too important. As I said, this road is not easy.

A great friend of mine, a very true spirit called Scott, reminded me, when I was whining to him about some minor difficulties with people through work that I had chosen this. He reminded me that I do walk this road alone, and it is mine alone to walk. Others may be beside me – my family, real family, select friends – supporting me, even cheering me on, but ultimately this is still my own contract, my own journey. My own responsibility activated the moment I chose to acknowledge it.

And I accept that responsibility. For it is my responsibility to show you the amazing gift you already have within. To heal yourself. To heal others.

So what about you? Do you know yet? Have you felt it? What is it that your contract entails?

Good news! I have some answers for you. Some I know to be true. But the truest answers are within you.

First of all: what you don't need. You don't need a constant channeller. I know it was handy for me (actually it was bloody terrifying at first) but when a convenience becomes a crutch you're no longer on your right path. Things are changing rapidly on this planet of ours. The energy has shifted, accelerated and grown, and you have the singular ability to reach in and feel that energy, know it, and learn.

You don't need protection. Truly, there is nothing to fear in this. When a client gets on the table for the first time, I always tell them that if they are worried or frightened all they have to do is open their eyes and they're back again. Hundreds of clients later and not one has opened their eyes for fear.

You don't need a guru or a leader. No not even me. (You don't want to put me on a pedestal: I'd probably mistake it for a podium and start dancing.)

You already have a master. You! And that is what this entire process, known as life, is about: Mastery.

Mastery is that journey up the staircase we spoke of. It is not a door you go through. There is no arrival, as such. Going up that staircase, one step at a time, you are able to reach into and master the one thing on this planet that you can master; **You**. Mastery is the development of the tools within you, the gifts within you; so that you may own the role that you are here for. Reaching beyond the known, trusting the new calm in your heart, moving forward despite the fear and embracing who you truly are: in this you are the Master.

More people work in "healing", than are titled so. For some call themselves "clairvoyant", some call themselves "office staff", some call themselves "parents", and of course there are many more. As they recognize, invite and enhance their unique gifts, unbeknownst to them they each know Mastery. Each of these people, through their unique assets and role, bring about healing in others just in their day-to-day existence.

I know I honour the "masters" that assist me when I teach, or when I work, as I consider their role equally as important as my own. After all, people come to the course, sessions, program or conference, through those people. My task is to show you. Their task is to show you how to get there, so that you *can* be shown.

Mastery runs on all and many levels, not least of all on a conscious level. It isn't just about the academic, or the spiritual, the scientific or the physical, or any particular level, awareness or point. It's about *all* of them. The rudimentary and the divine.

We as humans need to master and learn from all elements. After all we still have to survive here too, don't we? Mastering the crude and superficial can be necessary too.

In this process of healing, all levels are an asset. You will, as I have suggested, reach different people at different levels, but most essential in this, is how you reach you. What may seem rudimentary is no less essential in becoming the person you are becoming.

"Direct all forces with the hand of a master, and so bring them into harmony with the casual energy and source of all things."

James Allen

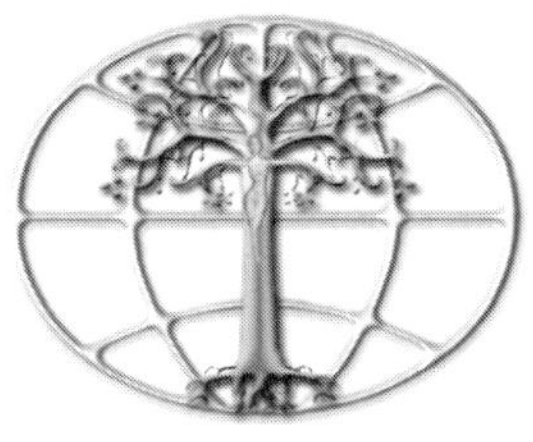

The "What"

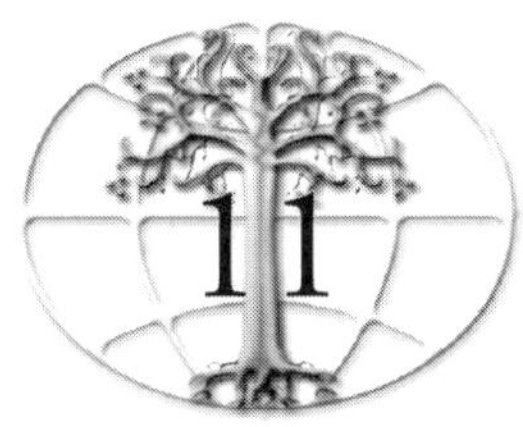

"He who lives largely in the ten earthly elements, and who is blind and deaf to the spiritual verities, will find no attraction in the doctrine of self-surrender, for it will appear to him as the complete extinction of his being; but he who is endeavouring to live in the ten heavenly qualities will see the glory and beauty of the doctrine, and will know it as the foundation of Life Eternal."

James Allen, author As a Man Thinketh

The Session Experience

What they feel at this end.

The client experience, physically and mentally, at this end is fairly much what you would expect at this stage. The very nature of acquainting, or reacquainting their body with these frequencies means that similarly to what you feel in the transference of the frequencies, between your own hands or through your body, they will feel in transition too.

Clients often feel a breeze around the table, or may sometimes refer to movement, as if someone was walking or "rushing" around the table.

Some feel a lifting or pulling sensation on a specific part of their body, usually an area that required attention such as an injury, deformity or affected organ. Many of the clients that refer to this particular sensation experience it around the abdominal area.

There are variations of tingling, buzzing, something akin to pins and needles, hot or cold areas.

A common recollection from many in session is a warm pressure on, and somehow *in*, their chest, right above the heart. Perhaps this too is related to the "ease" that so many come to know.

Some clients say they can feel where my hands are, even though I'm not touching them at all. And more often than not I don't actually have my hands close to the body at all. Some feel heat from them. Others refer to a concentrated breeze, like a cool beam touching them. And speaking of touching…

In this form of healing, which is a *hands-off* healing technique, clients often do report feeling physically touched by someone. Many clients get off the table saying, "Did you touch my shoulder?', and "Did you poke my chest?" "Were you holding my foot? Someone was holding my foot the whole time." All of this warrants a huge restraint from sarcasm on my part. Of course I don't go about prodding clients while they're supine on the table!

Who touches them? Who indeed. Some refer to them as guides, or angels, but for now, and for my sake, let's call them *entities.* No, not alien entities, or poltergeist, ghosts or any other entity we are conditioned to fear.

They are Spirit. They are also friendly (there is an understatement!). Intuition and instinct tell me that they pose no threat, and for the most part no pressure. There is absolutely no doubt in my mind that they play a crucial part in the client's journey or experience. Much of the presence in the room is there for the individual on the table. Each session brings about a unique unfolding, and the spiritual party tasked to assist in that is bound to be equally unique. What the client knows in experience on the table may explain this more.

What they see at their end

Yvette, in her ninth year of suffering from the disease of Lupus, came in for a second session. What follows is her account of what occurred during her experience in session.

"At first I saw colours, kind of slowly spattering against a glass just in front of my eyes, and then spiralling away, one at a time; beautiful colour, restful in its action. And I was thinking this is so lovely, and I felt so warm and comfortable for the first time in years that I was a little angry when I seemed to slip right through the colour and away from it."

"I don't remember getting there, if I did travel there, all I recall is gliding into an infinite multicoloured field of what I thought was tissues. Down a cleared pathway through the field a woman waited for me. She had long dark hair, symmetrically wavy. Her dress was, I think, a cream colour, but somehow shone. It was a simple dress that went to the ground, sort of medieval in shape, but not decorated, even though beautiful.

"Her face shone brightly too, so I couldn't really see her face. And I knew, somehow, that this was the most beautiful of women. And I knew she was smiling at me. I didn't see her mouth move, I didn't hear her actually speak but I knew she was talking to me. Her name had a "Sch" sound, but I couldn't understand it."

"Her greeting was warm, and as I approached her, it was like my heart thrust toward her, my chest swelled, and I felt overcome with emotion. Everything at once: sad, happy, joy, peace, shame, all welled inside me until I felt I would explode. And I was crying and laughing and smiling all at once."

"She lead me through the pathway of what it turned out was flowers, not tissues. Flowers I'd never seen, in colours I hadn't seen, and the smell… sweet and floral, but more like food, than flower. We walked together, she was saying something to me, and then she turned and faced me, and clearly I heard her, 'Yvette, are you ready to heal from this disease?' I told her that Melissa had already asked me this question, and, yes, I was ready."

"Then suddenly I felt dreadful, and doubled over with the pain (*during her session Yvette suddenly sat up and retched, then quietly lay back down*). I vomited on the pathway, but to my horror it wasn't fluid. Black crawling creatures, like spiders were being spewed upon the earth at my feet and as they ran and scattered, they disappeared into the ground."

"Shaking and afraid I looked up at her. She said, 'You are healed. You are free of this disease.' She indicated that we continue on together and we went further into the field of flowers. And the next I knew, Melissa was touching my shoulder and smiling at me."

Four weeks later, Yvette's doctors confirmed she had in fact gone into remission. I recently received an email from Yvette telling me she and her husband were expecting their first child. She did heal herself… with the help of a friend.

This is the part of the book that could blow you away. Those that are, shall we say, more conservative out there, or at least more conventional, are probably ready to dump this book in the garbage. Take it from me; I do know how this element of this healing process challenges your belief system. If I didn't know this to be true from experience, I, too, may very well be scoffing at this myself.

When you hear the term "New Age" it's a bit like hearing the term "Amway", isn't it? You can't help but cringe, even though you don't really know why. I've come to the conclusion that it's actually for the same reason: because there have been some unethical imbeciles out there misleading people and misrepresenting what they claim to so stoutly believe in.

So when we hear about angels, and guides, Pleiadian

masters, and spiritual entities, it can be hard to resist saying, "Yeah, whatever." A very gifted clairvoyant woman, Faye, was doing a reading for me, but when she said, "I'm going to use the cards now," I surprised myself with my own level of cynicism, when I thought, "Great. Here comes the tarot!" It turned out to be just a normal deck of cards. And sure enough there are people out there, reading this right now, and saying, "I thought this book was about *healing*! What is this crap?"

In all these years of my working with these frequencies, hundreds of clients have walked through the doors, and a number of great teachers and friends have come along throughout the journey as well. But from the very start, I have had four friends assisting in the process of facilitating healing who have always been consistent: A women, two gentlemen, and an animal…all in Spirit. Occasionally, apparently I too, make the odd appearance. I'll try to explain that too.

Yvette described one of the women very well, with her dark hair and gentle yet firm demeanour. She appeared to clients within the first few days of my starting in this. Occasionally, for some reason, people will suddenly open their eyes during the session and later tell me that as I was on one side of the table, she was on the other.

The first gentleman is wonderful. Warm and generous and joyous, you feel safe in his care. My children, who of course can see him clearly and quite effortlessly (unlike their mother), call him "Santa". He is tall and slender (unlike Santa) and has a white beard and white hair. People describe him as a wizard, with his long robes and beard, and every now and then a *Lord of the Rings* fan comes in and calls him "Gandalf". He is easy to visualize, isn't he? Coincidentally, his name does have a "g" sound to it.

Another gentleman started to appear about a year after I had started working in this, and initially I called him "the Overseer". Authoritative in some way, he felt like the boss. The first time he came in during session I knew he was there and in my heart I could see his image clearly. I soon after referred to him as the "blue lady". He isn't blue, he is actually garbed in blue, a rich sort of royal blue, but as Yvette described it he also "shines" so it's not a solid colour. His dress is similar in shape to the dark haired woman (hence, the blue *lady*), but he also has a head dress/ hat upon his head.

His demeanour is quite different to the others. As yet he has never communicated with the clients, although they do see him. He does communicate with me, and usually appears when I am learning: in a trying situation with a client, trying something differently or something new has come through, hence, why I call him the overseer. He too is generous, a little more serious and you feel his strength. He's quite extraordinary.

The animal… well, I don't really want to give this one away. She is big, feline and female. If you were to see her you'd know it. Wonderfully maternal, fiercely protective, you feel her leading the way. There's no mistaking this one's presence. I was astonished to discover, only relatively recently from Scott Alexander King, who works in animal shamanism, that she is also my "totem" animal. When children see her they have no fear of her and some during their session even ride upon her back, yet adults usually respond at first with terror.

Children see any number of animals whilst in session, and, according to the kids, a lot of the animals talk. Not the primary feline that I mentioned earlier – apparently she guides them but doesn't talk. But giraffes, zebras, bears, swans and many more, appear to the kids then somehow are still there, but no longer as the animal they originally showed themselves to be.

No, they are not of this world. No, they are not evil. My best description, my heart tells me, they are angels. And unlike any angel I ever been taught about. There are no choirs singing and I've seen no wings. There is no benign smile or superiority complex. They also can get impatient or a little demanding which doesn't fit the traditional description either really. More than that you feel their concern and caring and their pleasure at being part of it: they are there to assist in the process.

We've been conditioned to fear spiritual entities, haven't we? Movies, books, television shows, and now many publications make a fortune from that same educated fear in us. It's worked on me too. I confess I'm glad I'm not a medium. The "I see dead people" thing isn't for me. Since working in this I have seen a few "ghosts", but only a few, and thankfully, I know a few people that can help them out.

When I started this work, I joked with friends that I was the "reluctant gifted". Soon after the joke changed to; "I founded the club of the Reluctant Gifted". Some very well known psychics, healers, and mediums, amongst others, have joined this club! While the task in healing is simple, it isn't always easy. Even as things have progressed, and science converges into the spiritual, this is still well outside the square.

Of course, the greater source (God) knows that as humans in duality, fear is one of our constant and essential challenges. I assume that is why some people claim to see me whilst in session. In two different ways…

Sally, a young woman in the midst of a breakdown, was in session, when in her words, "I was shown a huge gold door and told to go through it, but I was scared. When I moved toward it, the door split open, turning into two doors that swung open. And *you* (Melissa) stood inside the room. It was like you were under a spotlight, but the light was somehow moving and sparkly…and I knew I would be okay."

I was at this end, I assure you, conducting the session. This has happened a number of times, different each time, but apparently I am there. My perspective is that perhaps in order to overcome their initial fear, they use an image people are more comfortable with, and in some cases that's me.

The other way I appear, is as I mentioned before, some

people for no reason they know of, suddenly open their eyes whilst in session and look at me. Many times, when they describe it to me after the session, clients have all used exactly the same words to describe it, "I was looking at you, but you looked different. Still I knew it was you."

When I said there was a spiritual element in this form of healing, I'll bet this is not what you were expecting. Even today, as I write, there are people out there who are thinking less of me for mentioning the Spiritual. There have been some scientists, in the face of this element, who chose to abandon researching and trying to understand this process. Downright insulting as they hurried out the door, I was left wondering… if they were *real* scientists surely they would embrace a challenging unknown.

After all, the greatest discoveries in science aren't those found in the moment when someone cries "I've got it!" Instead it's usually when someone is gazing into the galaxy or perhaps into the realms of the microscope, and they'll murmur to themselves, "Hold on. That's weird…"

Some people have been audacious enough to actually accuse me of "copping out" of responsibility of the healings, using the spiritual element as a cover, just in case nothing happens and there isn't a healing! Oh ye of little faith.

There is an incredible spiritual element that is communicating freely through these frequencies. Incredible, beautiful, rich and all love.

Not everyone experiences the session like this. Not everyone will see someone, let alone speak to someone or have such a profound journey that they are actually told they are healed. Some people just see colours, some just feel buzzing or heat or pressure, and yes, some do go the full gamut. Some are so caught in fear or ego, that despite the opportunity, they miss the real experience altogether.

A chiropractor came to me, who held a position uppermost in the hierarchy of a devout Christian-based church, with no other purpose than to waste over an hour of my time calling me a sinner (as if I hadn't heard that before!). He had been most insistent that he see me, and had come querying what and how I was doing what I do, but if I moved physically within a couple of yards of him he physically flinched. When I tried to explain and answer his questions, I offered it to him to feel the frequencies around his hand. At first he said, yes, use my right hand. Then, "No, no, no, I'm right handed, no, use my left hand. No, on second thoughts, don't touch me! Don't touch me! I don't want you to contaminate my spirituality!"

I should have resisted, but I didn't. "If your faith is so true, how can it be contaminated? Unless, of course, *you've* chosen contamination?" Fear: A many auspice thing. I tell you, it took some effort to kick this guy out, considering how fearful he was. But I managed it.

Just for future reference; if I ever have the privilege of facilitating a session for you, please don't try to impress me with a pre-arranged tale of what happened. I know it sounds strange, but people have done it! The only thing I see happening from divulging to me a farcical tale is a loss of experience for the person telling it. They'll be telling it to me in detail, text book true, and all I can feel is sadness at their loss. They were so busy trying to impress an ordinary individual at this end, that they missed an extraordinary journey into themselves.

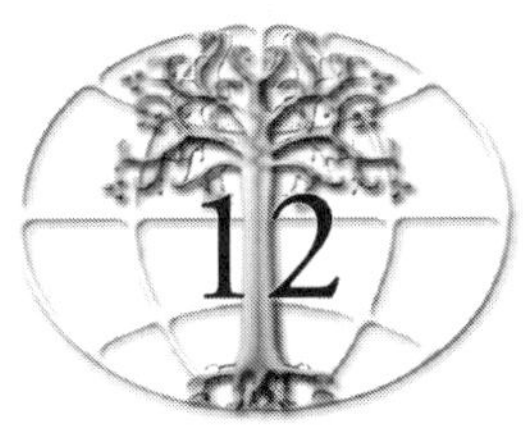

"I believe God is in me
As the sun is in the colour and fragrance of a flower
- the light in my darkness, the voice in my silence."
Helen Keller

Spiritual

God. Inside and out.

In a growing population of several billion individuals around the globe, more than ninety-five percent of them believe in some form of higher power. Of this group, more than half refer to that higher power as "God".

During the procedure of my own Axial Initiation™, while I was on the table, I came to know God (insert your comfortable title here: Spirit, universe, Life, light, etc) as I had never known God before. I came to *know* God, not *believe* in Him. And what I came to know was so astonishingly bigger and better than I had ever known, or had been lead to believe. I couldn't have "known" this intellectually; it had to be experienced because experience is, for a human, the only adequate language in which to know this. I am honoured when complimented by people who tell me that I am quite articulate, and yet the vocabulary I have available is utterly inadequate to describe this knowledge.

During my Axial Initiation I recognized within me a memory, and a *knowledge*, and suddenly, consciously I found myself belonging to a minority group.

I have known people who had believed in nothing beyond what they knew in the immediate from sensory feedback, that all went dark when you died and that's it.

I have known people who *suspected* that there might just be something out there.

I have known people who *did* believe, wholly knowing a faith in their heart, and living within that belief.

And then there was us, the minority: those who *knew*. Those who owned a knowledge held within the heart, honest and absolute. In the last decade I have watched this minority group undergoing such a ground swell!

You may recall, during my Axial Initiation, that I arrived at "God's blue". Not a destination but an emotion, all encompassing and unfettered. Love. I despise calling it love, because love as we know it is but an inkling of what I knew at the "blue".

Love. From me, that is what God really is, in everything. Real love. And when you feel it, it takes you to the very brink, almost truly overwhelmed, where you feel you cannot physically take any more, that you will blissfully explode. This love, it has substance, consistency. It has a viscosity and a movement that you cannot see, I doubt you could measure it, but it is rich and thick with ecstasy. Your heart swells singing amid recognition as it arrives. We have, all of us, known this love before.

The "Higher Source", a term that has decorated our collective conscience for some time, is finally being recognized within its true home.

Within.

The fact that your body will recognize these frequencies, remember them, in and of itself is showing you that this higher source can be found in you. This complete love. Yes, your heart knows this absolute love! Reach out and embrace your belief, for when you do so a connection is formed, a vibratory resonance comes to be. And you will know contentment unlike anything you've known before.

When people come into my rooms for a healing session, I can make no guarantees as to what gets healed. But the one thing I can assure you of is this: You will get off the table with a new contentment in your heart. I used to explain it as, "Your heart will just feel good", until a client said it beautifully, "It's like your heart has a big *ease.*"

During session, whether you are conscious of it or not, you know this love. That knowledge does not leave your heart, either. Where that new knowledge allows you to go is incredible. I have seen hundreds of clients achieve amazing things.

More and more you can understand why I consider what I do, a "healing initiation".

I know it sounds clichéd, "God Is Love", and for that I do apologise. So much I wish I could hand this feeling to you, so then you can understand the language of experience. In session, as a facilitator, I guess I have the privilege of doing exactly that.

Carl Jung used the word "*self*" for the god image in the psyche, the god within. If we can go within and find that image that has meaning to us, and honour our relationship with it, we provide the means for the spiritual impulse to express itself. Your existence can now go beyond the boundaries of simple conscious human existence.

First, let us draw the distinction between being "spiritual" and being "religious".

God is spiritual. Man is religious.

Religious doctrine is the instrument of man. Structured religions, their rules, regulations, and obligatory repentance are designed, drafted and implemented by man.

You know of my past, my upbringing ensconced in

Catholic and Christian churches. The root values of Christianity, drawn from the commandments, are not so original as the Christian faiths may hope to believe. Nearly all religions house a base in similar values.

Viewing this from a broad perspective, you have to consider that at the very core of us, the human being, we *do* know what is true and what is right. I mean leaders in all churches have put in place, both in scripture and enforced idealism, almost identical doctrines at the very core of their religious structures. Yes, we could all become critical of how true any church may be to those values, or question how they interpret those values in order to justify their actions. Let's not.

How religion has changed throughout the ages! What an incredibly secure format it once provided politically. Believing in it's own righteousness it has declared death sentences in its name. Instrumentally and functionally it has adorned us in grace and beauty, for primarily there was always Spirit (God). And in delusions of supremacy, religion has taken us to wars in far-flung places all across the globe. Even to that most dangerous and volatile environment: the dinner table.

The Dead Sea Scrolls abound with issues that could cause quite a dilemma for those higher religious leaders who are privy to them. Public exposure of such documentation the wisdom held within could indeed cause drama. For in no small way do they put question to the malleable manipulation of Christian values and how they were delivered to the common man. Of course, this type of manipulation is not mutually exclusive to Christian-based religions either.

I choose not to go into a debate about "Chinese whispers", inaccurate scripture and whether or not literal interpretation is appropriate.

In my very Indigo way I will attempt to share my definition of "religion": **Religion is a structured doctrine, assimilating or at least appearing to have a base in faith.**

I would give you an "official" definition from the

Macquarie or Oxford dictionaries, but they seem a little undecided themselves. My definition of "spirituality":

Spirituality; it is within. Spirituality is the peace and the power within you. It comes from the heart, lives within your true memory and is all that is whole, true, and love. It's what empowers us make the hard decisions for the greater good. It enables us to move forward when all duality of humanism cries against it. It lives within. It resonates without.

It has no recognition of how many times your butt sat in the front pew, or for how many Sundays you were there. True spirituality keeps no record, imparts no judgment, and offers no superior recognition. The only house it requires is you. Spirituality is not about faith; it's about belief and truth…at the very core of you.

Every time you come to the necessity for belief, you will be challenged with self doubt. Have you noticed that? Every now and then, in a moment of fatigue or fluctuating hormones, just like you I doubt myself. At these times, Spirit doesn't abandon you, *belief* does.

Two plus two equals four.

It doesn't matter whether you believe it or not. It does.

Some things just are.

Deep within you remember. And when you do, you will believe.

Believe. Trust, and believe.

There is no lower human being than I. There is no higher human being than I.

I no longer believe in a God that points the finger in judgment, and, if I don't keep my merit points up, sends me to Hell. Trust me, if God were going to strike people down, I'd be long gone. God probably doesn't need to judge us, for we humans judge each other, every day.

My children, ever my teachers, have no concept of "different", and certainly no fear of it. Because of the issues that

Jack lives with, we spend a lot of time attending various appointments at the Royal Children's Hospital in Melbourne. This hospital houses the best doctors and paediatric specialists from all over the world, so you tend to see some of the most extreme patient cases there as well.

We were in the elevator one day when a little girl and her mother got in. Clearly this little girl had cancer, and looked terrible, particularly as they had had to put the plug for all her drips into her head. People were avoiding looking at this little girl. Colby, my four-year-old daughter, on the other hand walked over to her and took her hand in silence. Then, when the elevator door opened, the two of them smiled at one another and raced out of the elevator, giggling. Her mother was driving the pole with all the drips and pumps on it and was forced to race after them.

A sixteen-year-old boy with severe level of Cerebral Palsy was in the day surgery waiting area with us. An attractive kid, but he had such a severe level of athetosis (spasmodic muscular ticking and jerking) that he had to be strapped quite dramatically to his chair to keep him somewhat still. People wanted to stare, but were afraid to make eye contact with him in case he spoke to them. Teagan, my youngest daughter, two years old at the time, sashayed over, clambered up, sat in his lap, and started talking with him. Why not? After all he *was* sitting down (in his wheelchair!). Teagan had that two year old semi-babble with every other word making sense and was cheerily prattling on. After a while, I heard him say to her through his smile, "You have worse speech than me!"

There is no lower human being than I. There is no higher human being than I. Believe it.

This gift of healing requires belief and will at the same time bring about belief. Each time God validates someone with a healing, it actually validates the individual, not a religion and not some protocol. From within.

Science and the Spiritual are converging. It had to happen. That's the evolutionary life; to redraw on all assets and shift forward uniformly.

Where are these frequencies coming from? From the Universe. Be it God, Life, Higher self, whatever you choose to call it. Recent findings in the study of the human genome have lead to the discovery of "gaps" in the DNA code, once known as junk. The extraordinary community of scientists that have converged upon the breakdown of the genome have come to believe, from the small deciphered amount we now recognize, that these gaps in the DNA code actually might contain the memory of the complete human.

Encompassing the spirit within, the mapping of the structure of this life, the predetermined challenges, the whole of who you are, beyond our conscious knowing, the memory of last experiences, maybe even past lives, the very imprint of the plan you had in place when you came to be here.

These gaps aren't "visible" to us yet. Already we have discussed that some of the DNA matrix is yet to show itself. Exciting isn't it?! Science and the Spiritual are converging.

As they need to in the inevitable evolution of the human race.

Where are these frequencies coming from? Well...where do you experience them from? Gather the knowledge that speaks loudest and truest to you, from every corner of the spiritual globe, and from that, all one can ask is that you trust in your own personal belief system.

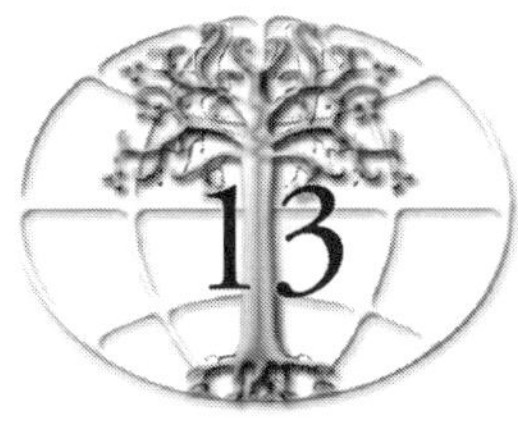

"Love adds a precious seeing to the eye"
William Shakespeare

Communication

I had received a call that was intriguing. Two women, Mary and Regina, both in their late forties, wanted me to go to them so that I could work on both of them. They had found my name in an article in a magazine that I didn't even know I was in (turned out there was an article). They needed me to go to them at night (they claimed they worked) and they couldn't come to me as they didn't drive. But they desperately needed me to go to them, as soon as possible; in fact they would pay me double to go to them. But it was curiosity, not money that took me there.

I pulled up at a magnificent house that had to be worth millions of dollars. As I approached the front entrance I heard a strange hissing noise,

"Psst. Pssst! Melissa!" A woman was whispering to me from around the corner of the house. "Come around this way!" She anxiously gestured that I follow her.

As I rounded the corner, I asked, "Is everything all right?"

"Sshhh! Just come this way." I followed her.

Down the side of the house was an entrance that would have been the servant's entrance, and that's what we entered. I had barely set foot in the door and noticed that a massage table was already set up, when in a billowing flurry of wafting ethereal robes, the two women apparently raced one another to the table competing to see who could go first.

Already, of course, I was asking myself "What was I thinking"?

This was a single room, large and dark, furnished, and occupied by the ladies, two cats and a dog, a massage table covered in multiple rugs and a few lambskins (perhaps it doubled as an alter?) and many, many candles.

The ladies started telling me that I was not to leave the room and enter the house, that my "dark energies" must remain contained in this room. Bad news; my bladder was full. So they *blindfolded* me and told me I must "hold my breath" as I was led to a bathroom within the house. As soon as I returned to the room, the race was on again, with the two of them tearing across the room and this time managing to bowl the table over. Mature.

Mary said, "Fine! You go first, Regina. I think I'm going to channel anyway."

I know I was looking forward to it.

Mary sat down in a chair, her hands clutching the arms, feet flat with her legs apart, and preceded breathing coarsely and heavily.

I turned back to the table and gave Regina the run down then started the session. I was hoping for a quick one. They hadn't really called upon me for any specific physical issue, more for the experience. But of course, once I started working you could feel it all; a little tennis elbow here, some menopausal hormonal stuff there, a little work around the head, the thyroid, and more. I was working away, occasionally reaching down to pat the dog, who was sitting under the table, when all of a sudden I felt really uncomfortable, every nerve on edge.

Mary had been breathing heavily behind me, and I confess I hadn't noticed the absence of it. I turned to look at her, to find her staring at me, staring hard and cold, with both her hands up, palms facing me. She said, "You are not an angel." I doubt I showed any surprise at this announcement. All the same I was just sick of the melodrama at this stage, so using my scary Army voice (as my kids call it) I commanded, "Put your hands down, and take your seat."

She was completely taken aback and appropriately scared. Once she had regained her performance/composure, she chose to blame her little outburst on the Pleiadian masters channelling through her. Of course it was.

Regina's session was forty-five minutes. I have nothing nice to say about that. She got off the table, burst into tears, and told of the beauty and wonder of what she had experienced and she was genuine. She had the shakes and was somewhat overwhelmed. She sat upon the couch with a rug and the cats comforting her.

These women had paid double for me to be there, so Mary was next to the table.

Now you can imagine that "What am I doing here?" phrase was loud in my mind. What was I learning here? Patience (I'm still learning that one)? Tolerance? Regardless, I started the session.

Mary had been exposed to the frequencies as I had worked on Regina, so she took off fast. *Please let it be quick!* A knee injury of some sort, arthritis starting in her ankles, hormones again...From the outset I kept hearing the phrase "airhead". Initially I thought, fair enough. She'd certainly behaved as one. Again "airhead" and I thought, is this my subconscious? I'm not usually so insistent when I am derogatory; "airhead". So I asked, mentally, "What is it that you want me to know?"

The answer was very clear; "Call her "airhead"." I didn't *hear* it; there was no voice in my head, or my ears. It was like I suddenly knew the answer to a question I had never asked. The answer did not come to my mind, it came to my heart. And I just knew it. And what an answer!

Such communication had been coming to me before this, but seeds of doubt and blatant disbelief, not to mention fear, had convinced me that it just couldn't be. I didn't trust it. On this night, with this trying situation, the lesson was becoming very clear. But "airhead?"

I was thinking "I'm not saying that! How rude!" But I heard it throughout the session. "Call her 'airhead'." I finished her session, and tears ran down Mary's face. Apparently she had been chastised for her earlier behaviour (go Spirit!). And she had been healed.

I sucked up my courage as I recounted my version of the session to her and said, "Mary, I wish I could say this so it doesn't sound so offensive, but I kept hearing the phrase "airhead" while I was working..." A new flood of tears coursed down her cheeks and the verbal flood soon followed. Her husband and all his family actually called her that to her face, and had done so for years. The hurt was deep and well worn. And a new lesson took hold within me.

Learning to listen. Trusting what I had come to know.

Listening

Remember Helen, my wonderful friend and business manager? She had been ill for a while, she had a cough that wouldn't go, and was really tired. She thought it was burnout (not from me! I promise). Of course, over a series of months I had worked on her, but I couldn't really find anything, and it didn't seem to make much difference. Out of nowhere, on Christmas Eve, she called me from her doctor's office.

They had found 67 cancerous masses in her lungs. She had six weeks to live.

Helen and I had met when she was dragged to me by a friend, as a client. The moment her friend left the room, she said, "I don't know what the hell I'm doing here. I don't need this." Always the start to an amazing session. Thirty minutes later, Helen started channelling while on the table. This had happened before, with other clients, but it was usually during an Axial Initiation. I guess Helen and I were both surprised on this day.

I was quietly working away when suddenly and loudly she said "Three months, four days. You can change this." The room had been silent, so really I was lucky to hear this over the thumping of my own heart! It was her voice, not the screechy, gagging stuff I had heard when people had channelled in the past, yet I knew it wasn't Helen speaking. I started to ask questions, and the voice answered. I was told what to do, that I must "enhance this", what to look for, and even not to drink red wine as post-cancer my liver cannot handle it (a fact proven at my brother-in-law's wedding). I was also told that 'this one', Helen, now knew her task.

After the session Helen told me that from the very start she had felt the need to speak but had fought it. She thought she had been coughing throughout the session as she continued to fight the urge to speak, but felt like she had a rock in her throat.

Helen effectively became my personal communication channel with Spirit. If I just didn't get it or understand it, couldn't clearly hear what was being communicated through me, I'd say "Helen? Would you mind?" She'd sit in her favourite recliner, I'd start to work putting her into session, and *they'd* start to chat. I'd ask questions, argue with them, they would instruct or direct and it was always interactive. A true gift.

Now I was to lose her. Sixty-seven cancerous masses, and

the moment I heard that, I knew she was leaving. Sure she gave lip service to fighting it but within a week it had spread everywhere. I was losing Helen, my friend, my manager, one of the most brutal teachers I'd had…it was like losing my mother. Her embrace meant more than most to me. I was desperate to learn how to embrace her after she had left.

I needed to learn communication.

A wonderful friend had invited me to a clairvoyant circle. While I had been invited to many different groups, for some reason this was the right one. The timing was bizarre! Before I went, I knew I would only go three times, despite their request for a two year commitment.

What an amazing group of people. My gratitude goes to them for the lessons, intense and soul-baring as they were.

My first night there, all of them did trance mediumship! All of them channelled, including my friend which was delightful if not entertaining to watch! Considering myself a mere onlooker, you can imagine my shock when they announced it was my turn! I was asked to perform psychometry. This is where they hand you a piece of jewellery belonging to someone else, and you try to read (clairvoyantly pick up information about the owner) from it.

I closed my eyes and a watch was placed in my hand. I opened my eyes, and the group leader said, "Okay, Melissa, now tell us if you get anything from it. Does it feel hot or cold? Do you see any colours?"

I had to be honest, "No, I'm sorry, none of that. But, I could I tell you about the person if you like." I added hopefully. He gave away nothing. "Okay, try that."

"How personal do you want me to get?"

He assured me he would stop me if I got too personal. So I told them about the woman that owned the watch, who at that moment was feeling utterly inadequate in the room, like everyone else was gifted but her (join the club). I had an image of the last time she'd known complete joy, and began to describe a time when she was only four or five in detail… a woman in the room started to cry; messy, heartfelt sobbing. I handed her the watch and some tissues, and turned to the group leader.

"That's all I got. I didn't see any colours or anything though. Sorry." I thought I had failed miserably.

Helen laughed so much when I recounted this session to her that we had to increase her oxygen. She said, "Mel! They asked you to crawl and you said, "Sure, let me just sprint off into the distance, and then I'll come back and crawl for you."

She then said, "Did you know who owned the jewellery before they gave it to you?" I told her when they suggested I do psychometry; I knew that the item was going to be that particular lady's.

Helen said, "Listen, Mel, listen! You *already* knew. So what is it you're trying to learn? You need to pause and *listen.*"

Apparently it's called claircognizance, to know the answers to things you never asked. Rather than box myself in, I think I may be "clair-all-of-it". Really, why limit ourselves?

During session I know a lot about the person on the table, both the physical attributes and more. Often I can also be privy to the spiritual mix that is with them, too. It seems to me, and this is only my theory at this stage, but it's like a build up of information as these frequencies travel through me. And then I know the answer to the unasked question. I quite often know what they experience on the table, and who visited in the room during the session, before they tell me. Just because I was there in the same frequency as I facilitated it, I guess.

We are told these frequencies are built on "light and information". *The Keys of Enoch; the Book of Knowledge* offered me a broader more precise explanation, regarding this communication: "*If man can work with the new Light inputs of higher orders of intelligence, he can begin to induce enzyme reactions with the combined alpha and delta levels of thought so as to direct his consciousness beyond his body."* Then, "*here the mind is able to go beyond the static levels (of the physical) into living divinity.*"

Directing consciousness beyond the physical body. Another lesson ensued…

Sometimes the reaction of a person in session can be dramatic to say the least. Completely unaware of it, at this end people will be crying, just sobbing, shouting out, cringing, curling into the foetal position…in short, people can look as though they are in distress. Early on I learnt not to interrupt them regardless.

One lady was crying and crying so I touched her shoulder gently, compassionately, only to have shouted at me, "What did you do that for?! You should have left me there!"

A few similar incidents later, and again as a woman sobbed upon the table, by sheer necessity I decided to try to figure out if she was alright. I wondered if I could somehow look at where she was. Almost accidentally I discovered that I could, briefly, project in to her experience and see what she was seeing. I hear nothing, it is all visual, and then only momentary. It was as if someone said, "Okay Mel, you can have a quick look then you're out of there! No loitering allowed."

The first time I actually managed it, I physically fell over next to the table. I had for a moment completely lost awareness of my own physical sensation. It could have been the shock too. But in that moment, I had seen or rather somehow known the incredible rapture that the client was experiencing. Extraordinary.

These days I try to be a little more subtle and definitely more refined in my projection. Communication is not my primary gift, not the spiritual kind anyway. One thing this group taught me is that we do all have the ability to do this kind of work. Both the psychic abilities, from the self, and the "clair-all-of-it", from the Source, from Spirit. Although there are some who are just astounding at it! It's not my primary gift, I'm here to tell you, but I'm getting better at it because I *am* listening.

On my second visit to the same clairvoyant circle I really upset them. I spoke to the spirits that were channelling through. The people in this group had no idea who I was or what I did (essential to the group purpose) so they were fairly taken aback when I started to converse with the spirits channelling through. I wanted to know who these spirits were, and why they presented in human emotion when they were in spirit. Were they stuck, such as a ghost, or had they brought themselves to such a level so that we, the stupidly human, could comprehend? So I started to ask questions, which those in spirit channelling happily answered, until I looked around at the scandalized faces of the physical group. Apparently my spiritual etiquette needed work. I wasn't revering the monologue.

One woman growled at me, "I thought you came here to *listen*? For someone *listening*, you seem to be talking a lot!"

I replied, "I came here to listen, not to *hear*. There is a difference. I am here to learn, not applaud." Honestly, I *am* an Indigo. It took *me* thirty years to finally realise not everyone thinks like me! Or that I don't think like anyone else.

When people channel on the table in session, it's instructional, but not authoritative. They help and teach and show and guide. They do tell me off for not taking care of myself enough, but never for my work. They also at the same time put me under pressure!

The third time I was there, as a wonderful entity whom I had met before was channelling through, I thought I would just quietly "feel" him. I was sitting right next to the man channelling, so I gently projected into this spirit. The spirit in question stopped speaking mid-sentence, turned his partner's body toward me, smiling, and announced, "I would continue but my friend here is feeling me." Nothing untoward I assure you!

He asked what I was feeling and I answered honestly and we talked about it. The scandalized faces were once again agape as he said, "They do not understand. But the work you are doing is important and you must go forward. We will help Helen. We are ready to take her hand now. She will not be alone for a moment."

Six weeks to the day from the diagnosis, Helen went Home.

In my experience true learning, and hence wisdom, comes in the silence as you go about processing the input you take on. It is in this place that true communication occurs. Those moments of quiet, for me, stand alongside my client sessions, as the greatest classroom of all.

Unlike me, do not wait until you are in dire straits to learn communication in whatever form it suits you. Reach out to Spirit, to your Higher Self, so that it is familiar. Practice it regularly, wherever you can, whenever it suits, until it becomes involuntary and readily accessible. Recognize that communication is made so much more difficult when you are emotional, or tired, and trying to develop the art of listening within will get ugly if you start from a place of distress.

Allow me to quote exquisite verbiage from Deepak Chopra:

"*Spirit whispers to us through the gap between our thoughts and the slightest sensation in our body. This is why spending time in silence is so important. When we think of healing as the return of the memory of wholeness and wholeness as body, mind, spirit and environment, we begin to understand why we must learn to quiet our minds.*"

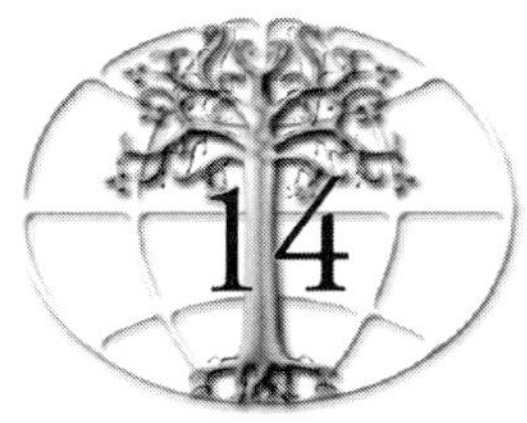

Be patient toward all that is unsolved in your heart…
Try to love the questions themselves…

Do not now seek the answers,
which cannot be given
because you would not be able
to live them.

And the point is,
To live everything.

Live the questions now.
Perhaps you will then
gradually,
without noticing it,
Live along some distant day
into the answers.

Rainier Maria Rilke

Let's Talk About You.

You are a never-to-be-repeated value in this universe.

I dare you to go and look at yourself in a mirror. I dare you. To honestly look upon yourself, faults and strengths intact, is one of the hardest things you can do, and as such most people will never really do it. But you can. Look at the wonder of your unique and exquisite self. You are gifted. You are. Kryon in his channelling refers to you, the human in lesson, as "*the exalted one*", for the courage and love you demonstrate while in lesson on this planet.

You are a never-to-be-repeated value in this universe.

You came here, to this world, with a diverse and unique range of gifts. You came intact, with them already within you. It takes the unfolding of your own journey for you to remember that they are there, in wait. The unfolding of this journey will lead you to stepping up to the contract and the plan you wrote prior to arriving here.

You are a never-to-be-repeated value in this universe.

You are reading this book, right now, because you have started to remember, started to acknowledge the purpose for which you came. And you have started to reacquaint yourself with the incredible healing ability within.

You have my heartfelt congratulations! What you are doing right now is crossing a line. The starter's pistol is probably ringing in your subconscious ear as you continue to read, because you have, indeed, entered a new realm in your own existence.

Having read all of this, you aren't really surprised, are you? Initially you probably got a little sarcastic about yourself, and said "Yeah, right!" But deep within, somewhere deeper than a place of ego or pretence, you knew it to be true when you read it.

"Deeper than a place of ego" is exactly what we're talking

about here. The constant battle of "having one foot, firmly placed, on either side of the veil", as Kryon again, so succinctly puts it, can leave us floundering in self doubt. You want to be logical, to prove what is happening, and not hear that little voice in the very back of your mind saying, "mental illness is starting now".

There is true beauty in the duality of being human, in the struggle of being human and existing adequately as such (for we *are* human and need to survive), and of being connected in unprecedented depths to the "other side of the veil", to the Source, as we go through the lesson, or the journey, that is this life.

These frequencies are awakening that imprinted but until recently denied to you, memory of your exact role and purpose. These frequencies, born of light and information, can, will and should do exactly that.

This new energy has come to this planet with purpose. There are no accidents here. For *you* have come to this planet with purpose too.

This is why this is "A Healing Initiation."

A thousand times you'll read and hear it from me that the physical healing is often the least of it. I have watched it happen for hundreds of clients, clients who have walked out without the cancer they walked in with, where the physical healing of body was simply the start of that individual's personal evolution.

More dramatically again is what occurs for the individual during the process of Axial Initiation™. The purpose of this procedure is to realign and reconnect the communication matrix within the individual, thus re-establishing connection through the axiatonal and meridian lines of the human energy anatomy. Whatever your gift is, your purpose, your role, this procedure enhances and reacquaints you with it. For many it is the first conscious recognition of their life "contract" or purpose… as it was for me.

It is such an awesome personal transition, truly sacred, that as the facilitating instrument implementing an Axial Initiation™ you can feel almost like you're intruding. Every time I undertake this procedure for another individual, triggering this evolutionary transition, it is astoundingly unique, and always just plain astonishing.

These frequencies are opening a door, just a crack at this stage that we are welcome to walk through as we became more capable of doing so. The avenue open to you now may not be exactly in the direction you thought it might be. You may need to reverse up a little first. For you need to go within, before you can give without.

A warning: you're about to feel a little uncomfortable.

Because the duality that it is to be human at this time, on this planet, as these incredible evolutionary shifts occur, dictates that you be uncomfortable at recognising your true potential. We are not yet in a position to fully recognise the spirit within us, but we have, as a biological population, started to. As the spirit within becomes more obvious the shackles of physical humanity begin to expand and we can no longer live with the safe and comfortable pretence that we are all there is in the universe.

Self doubt creeping in again? Surely you aren't that important, right?

Where you are right now is exactly the right moment, and the right place for you to cross the line and become all you were meant to be. The timing, despite what you may be thinking, couldn't be more appropriate. All the things that you ever will be or ever were are wrapped up in the potential of this very moment: your "now".

It doesn't matter how old you are, or what has happened in the past, mistakes you made or opportunities you feel you missed. I'm asking you not to worry about why you haven't come upon this sooner. You are right now exactly where you're meant to be.

Some of you are angry at me for saying this. Some of you are in such a tortured place, there is no way you would have consciously chosen your circumstances yet your heart knows I am writing truth…Every decision you have made, and every decision that was made for you, has put you exactly where you are now. It's that responsibility thing that challenges most, when you are facing the idea of those decisions that were made for you…Life can do that, can't it? Know that if you don't make the decision, Life will make it *for* you, and then we're stuck dealing with circumstances we would never have selected. Not making a decision, procrastination, is a decision in itself.

So what about your past? All that you've been through, and done? The past is gone.

The past is just old information. To live there serves no real purpose, other than guaranteeing a constant state of discontent. Who needs that?!

Regardless of what your past holds, *it doesn't hold you…* unless you let it. Don't let it. There is nothing that existed in the past that cannot be corrected now. In fact, I challenge you to look at the horrors that may reside back there and be grateful for them. For you would not be here, right now, reading these words, had those things not happened. It made you who you are right now. Actually, *you* made you who you are right now. Well done! Remember, there is a plan, and it is a plan of your making. Your future is of your making also…

The future is as yet undetermined, but it will be determined by you. So in its undetermined present state, treat the future like the past; let it go. You are so much more powerful than you know! The decisions you make in this moment, as situations arise in the present moment, and how you choose to deal with them are essential elements in your future. Where you allow your mindset to take you is drafting and designing your future. The future is yours.

Yesterday is gone. Tomorrow is undetermined. Today,

now, is what you have.

The fact that you are reading this book, right now, means that this is the right time for you to plant one of your feet a little more firmly on the "other side of the veil." Actually, already you were in the process of doing this when you picked up this book. For some of you, this is where the battle within the duality starts to rise, for fear is a major element in the battle. For those of you still shocked that I ruined it all by mentioning "spirituality" apropos the astounding ability to heal, my advice: forget it and let's go forward.

This is a journey. And you need to view it as a journey, not as an "arrival". Instead from this moment on, you can look upon this life as an ascending staircase, not a doorway: there is no arrival as such. There will be a gradual unfolding, and as you grow and ascend a little higher, taking ownership of each step up, you learn a little more and grow a little wiser. One day you will look back and realize how far you've come. And in such moments, the time will come when you go from success, to significance.

One of the hardest things for you to accomplish throughout your journey is letting go of old outmoded, preconceived thought patterns and habits. Humanity as a whole, as well as individually, is still trapped in half truths and concepts that originated thousands of years ago. The paradigms that we have been brought up in, in all areas, spiritual, religious, education, relationships, family, etc, and each so different for each of us, require us to now discard them with each lesson learnt, each stage of the journey completed.

In order to go forward as a species, as an individual, to continue on the ascension, we have to go beyond the traditional paradigms and boundaries of science, religion and spirituality. In doing so, we inadvertently commune and advance the process of greater evolution.

Already you have seen it through my eyes, and through the story of my journey to date; the constant flow in lesson, the gaining of wisdom, the recognition of knowledge that I was born to pass on. You've seen, by walking a distance through my life that experience itself can be the key to release from *a* life, into *your* life.

In your heart you know who you truly are and you always have. That is you! No, you are not delusional. Could it be that this is what you are here for? Are you feeling compelled to move forward with this extraordinary gift a part of you? Do you feel a calling to find out? Some will. Some won't. Somewhere, someone is. And all made the right choice.

In itself this process is where fear rises rapidly, isn't it? For to deal with these changing issues that are so primary in what we believe to be our make-up, is to step out of our comfort zone. A place none of us really likes to go. And in no small way. Even I, who love a challenge and live for the next adventure, always revel in the return to a comfortable place.

I don't want to write about fear because so many authors, wiser than I on this topic, have covered it so succinctly in so many different environments. I doubt very much that I can tell you much more about fear than you have heard before. But for that one person out there who hasn't heard this before, I am glad I did this for you.

Fear is essential to the human in lesson. Fear is a base emotional element giving birth to any number of other intrinsic and reactive emotions that add to the dramatic play that is life on this planet. Many of the emotions that you may have considered primary – anger, depression, envy, denial, and more – can be taken another level back to their base: fear.

To experience fear is to be human. Shackled and bound by biology, caught amid humanity, we are privy to the always unique, yet rarely predictable, mix of free will, emotion, ego, and the indomitable, ever-present, but not always acknowledged, you. When I speak of "you", I speak of the spirit you are, (despite that conscious memory of it doesn't seem at all present.)

As an Indigo, I see things in black and white. I see good and evil, right and wrong, yes and no, opposing elements creating balance. When you get right down to it, there is the ultimate balance, as a human, between absolute primary elements: the balance between love and fear.

When I first heard the term "shades of grey", I scoffed as any real Indigo would. It seems to me that sometimes those "shades of grey" people refer to are actually just a compromise on integrity. Only a human could believe there is an appropriate compromise on integrity! Rest assured, maturity has lent me a little more tolerance and patience with those shades of grey, not to mention a certain social requirement of acceptance, so that these days I don't scoff nearly so loudly as I used to.

Fear is not all negative. Fear is in fact a great tool for us in this life, for it allows us to set useful, even crucial, boundaries, aiding survival. The process is developed in the avoidance of reliving or experiencing pain, be it emotional or physical. That brief mental note you took, "I'm not going there again!" is the mapping of the perimeters that keep you comfortable, and often safe. Perhaps now for the first time you truly understand where the perimeters of your comfort zone are.

Combating fear? In simple terms, overcoming fear takes courage. Courage isn't doing something without fear. Courage is about doing something *despite* the fear. Courage is simply about overcoming the paradigms established in your own mind, and forcing that mindset to expand. It's about doing what you have to do *even though* your knees are knocking. In the action undertaken in courage, the comfort zone too does expand, but often, unfortunately, it is only a temporary alteration.

Particularly regarding the spiritual element of this gift, so easily I could have allowed fear to rule me. We are conditioned to fear the likes of ghosts, and spirits, communication and contacts from "worlds" not our own. And this fear is nurtured and marketed throughout all media in films, novels, television, etc.

The moment this gift hit me, so did the essential element of spirit, and "weird" stuff started happening to me and around me. Only days after my introduction to this I was taking a bath when little hand prints started appearing on the towel rail. I was alone in the bathroom, the towel rails were chromed and, like someone was gripping the rail, an impression of a hand would momentarily appear. It was a child's hand but to the naked eye there was no child. Then a little momentary condensation cloud would appear as if the child had blown breath upon the rail. For something this tangible I called in Andrew, who loved watching it and was most disappointed that when I left the bathroom, the child seemed to go with me.

Honestly, this sort of stuff freaks out the best of us, doesn't it? What I see these days, what I know to be true, in years past, I would have not only, seriously doubted, I would have quickly run from it! It took a complete re-education of the mindset and hence the paradigms that I had developed over the years, to overcome these pre-set fears. And so I overcome; for to not do so, would be to deny the potential within.

Indeed, there is a known antidote: Action cures fear. When taking action in the face of fear, sometimes it pays to think it through and sometimes its better not to think: Just jump in. Therein lay the power of free will and the challenge to rise above it. Helen Keller said of fear: *the best way out is through.*

Evil is only a decision away. So is true happiness. I remind you again, seek and live by your own truth as you know it. Become who you know you truly are, now. Every day. Share with us the amazing you.

Let us all see it.

The future is yours. Now is *your* time. And the potentials are awesome!

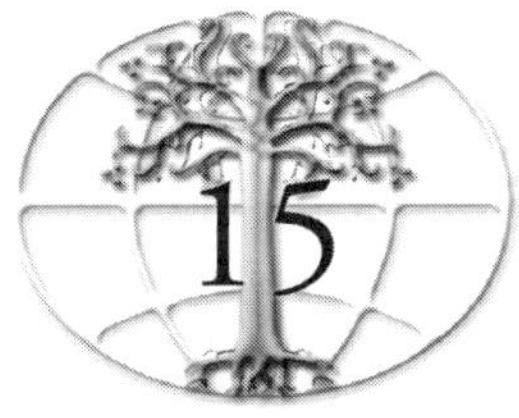

"Man is always the master. Even in his weakest and most abandoned state."
James Allen

The essential element of the mind

In this empowering gift clearly there is a divine spiritual element. Also, evidently we know there is a physical response, often appearing miraculous.

I know that I refer to your position as a "facilitator", as an instrument or tool through which these frequencies are transferred. In the explanation of these elements I recognize that I have separated, even displaced our selves from the process. Please don't be mistaken into believing that you are not essential in this process. You absolutely are. You are the frontrunner.

When it comes to utilizing these frequencies you are far more in control than you may believe. Actually you are far more in control of your life than you believe. The beauty of you being you is that you are the one thing over which you do have control on this planet. Of course, there are always those individuals who would believe they control more, but truly, this is only illusion.

You are far more in control than you may believe. The three essential elements in this consist of: the mind, the thoughts you allow to exist in your mind, and your personal mindset, all combined (yes, these three things are all different). Collectively, these three elements can make anything possible; absolutely anything is achievable, for you (Hands up, who saw the power of three there?) And now, with recognition of this amazing gift within you, there are no limits.

No, I am not contradicting myself. You are not in control of the healings. But, just as you are in control of how you respond and behave, you are in control of how you, as a facilitator, conduct these healing sessions. How effective those sessions are, and the possibility of how you grow, learn and go forward, is all within your control.

In *As a Man Thinketh*, James Allen writes, "*Of all the beautiful truths pertaining to the soul which have been restored and brought to light in this age, none is more gladdening or fruitful of divine promise than this – **that man is the master of thought, the moulder of character, and the maker and shaper of condition, environment, and destiny.***"

The power of the human mind, alongside the malleable element of will, is extraordinary.

The great thinking machine of the human mind is an extraordinary instrument through which any number of great events can and will take place. Your very life is your thinking and the result of your thinking processes. Yes, you are the product of your own thoughts. Put differently, your life is what your thoughts make it.

Wherever your thoughts are, your reality is. Your consciousness is the actual reality. The physical is only temporary. Your cellular structure, although a sacred vessel in itself, is only a place where the Spirit of your consciousness resides and you can take that spirit anywhere you want. You are infinite potential on legs, I tell you.

Thought itself? No one really knows what exactly thought is, other than it is some form of mental action. And yet, not unlike the unknown element of these healing frequencies, we see its manifestations everywhere. We see it in the expressions and actions of any single person, or even animal, any living thing really. To view thought in action, there are few better to look at than my own son's battle with his noncompliant body.

I mentioned earlier that Jack has a severe level of Cerebral Palsy. In addition Jack is also diagnosed beneath the umbrella of ASD (Autism). Jack's CP is spastic quadriplegia, so it affects his entire body. But nearly all of the tone, or spasticity in his body, is reactive tone.

To explain: When *we* move in any way, to pick up an object, jog across the street, scratch an ear, the brain habitually commands the body to do so without us ever really having to actually think about it. When Jack tries to move however, his brain communicates to the muscle groups needed for the movement, but then the muscle groups retaliate with a high level tone that seizes the muscles up. Jack then has to *remake* the decision to move and to *also* fight that spasticity throughout the entire movement. And this doesn't just happen in a gross motor movement like sitting up, reaching for something or walking, but also to speak, to eat, even to breathe. He's one amazing warrior.

Jack is a good looking little man and when he's propelling himself about in his fluorescent yellow wheelchair, he just looks like a kid that had an unfortunate accident. Not so long ago, we shared a brief incident which nicely demonstrates a *lack* of thought in action.

We were at the local bank and Jack was playing with the electric automatic doors. The doors would glide open and Jack would zip in and spin his wheels so the wheelchair would turn sideways, then stick his leg up and jam the doors open as they tried to close. Typical kid stuff, minus the wheelchair I guess. Unfortunately, this was the only entry into the bank. It was busy in there, and I was in the queue with my two little girls, chaos reigning as usual.

I looked over to gauge just how Jack was going in his automatic door challenge, and realized that people were waiting either side of the door to go through it. Some were amused at the antics, others were decidedly awkward in the face of a small disabled kid, but nobody would have the public audacity to ask him to move. So I called out, "Jack! Get out of the way!"

I heard him say, through his big smile "Sorry everyone," as he manoeuvred out of the way so they could pass. The lady in queue behind me was just itching to get my attention.

She said, "Is that your son?"

I looked at her, "Yes."

She said "What's wrong with him?"

I looked over at Jack again, and called out "Jack, what's wrong mate?"

He turned to look back at us, "Nothing Mum."

I looked this lady fair in the eye and said, "Nothing."

We all have the ability to use thought to our advantage, just not everyone does.

In your position as a human being walking this earth, the mind, alongside the heart, are your greatest allies. Because they are you, they are yours, and you do have control of them. In your position as a healing facilitator, the mind is a potent asset to you.

The heart? An essential.

One of my greatest pleasures in walking upon the planet is watching the interactions of people and where they allow themselves to go in that interaction. I study it in myself too. Ultimately, it all comes back to a single decision. Your **success** is only a decision away; your happiness, only a decision away,

contentment, a decision away. Your **ability** as a healer, as a person, as a parent, as a partner, only a decision away. Whether or not you live or die, is a decision away. And, evil, too, is only a decision away. The decision: will you cross that line?

Can you see this in yourself?

I'll bet you can remember a moment when you chose your reaction. Even in those moments when you had lost control emotionally, if you could be brutally honest with yourself, you'd admit that before you actually lost control, you made a decision to *let* yourself lose control.

It's not easy to have such control of your mindset, of your thought pattern. It's achieved through studying yourself honestly (*not* easy), and studying it a lot, and practicing until at last it becomes habit. The human in duality has to deal with gifts that masquerade as something other than a gift, such as ego, fear, envy, and the list goes on.

The power of the human heart and of the spirit within should not be underestimated either. How else could there still be extraordinary people, warm, generous, friendly people, around us? Perhaps I am naïve, or at least perceived to be, but I have faith in the beauty of the individual. I have faith that everyone has the potential to do the right thing.

We were brought to this planet with our will intact. Many religions have perceived the will of man as our downfall: the creator of sin, and the embodiment of evil. I don't believe man's will was without planning. Yet only in recent times has the human race evolved to the point where our destiny is now our own.

Through the strength of discovering the spirit within, we now have the ability to "co-create" and alter the future, to create our own future. The recent energy shift of this planet over the past few decades is evidence that we can co-create our future. Predictions from past prophecies that until the last few decades were remarkably accurate are no longer so, as the shift in the energy on the planet means that we have changed the outcome. Even the promised 2012 prophecies are far more positive and dramatically evolutionary, rather than the destructive mass annihilation once thought to be impending. Now the year 2012 shows itself to be more of a key turn in evolution, an emergence rather than annihilation.

Did one human change that future? Many did. Individually, amid their own unfolding journey, many chose to alter what seemed the inevitable in a smaller environment. Collectively, this is all-powerful.

It's my perspective that free will is one of the richest assets we as a human have. And particularly valuable when facilitating these frequencies.

Through practicing, various clients showed the need for an enhanced application of the frequencies. Originally I was challenged by the concept, as I had initially been taught to not "direct" the flow. But this wasn't "directing" as such, I wasn't beaming frequency into a certain point, but rather using a measured immersion of the body within the frequencies. Why? It created a more efficient flow, and less duel conflict between the physical experience and the far greater spiritual one.

It rapidly became clear, through sessions that we could quite easily use our body instrumentally, making the application of the frequencies even more efficient.

From the beginning of this, perhaps merely out of habit, I had been documenting and taking notes on what was happening for each client: what I had seen, what they had experienced, what I had "known" whilst working on them. I was quite conscious and aware of these frequencies changing as they evolved. As soon as I addressed the evolution of these frequencies *with intent*, they took off on their own, and palpably so! The frequencies were bigger, stronger, and even more all-encompassing; and not a little bit scary at times.

Over time, and again through experience, I've discovered

different needs in session with different clients, and as such, have found ways of meeting those needs appropriately; this in order to increase or decrease the flow, so as to keep the client as comfortable as possible at this end, and keep the distractions within their physical experience to a minimum. Not to mention the immense variance in how a session is conducted. What is most appropriate or affective, from doing a direct "hands on", to working an enormous charged field? What lies before you as you take this out there…? Let's just say, in this role you'll never get bored.

The human body, as the conduit vehicle or instrument, is far more pliable in the implementation of these frequencies, than first considered. Technique is in fact far more a part of the transference of the frequencies than I first acknowledged. In the healing process induced through the Quantum Bioenergetic balancing technique™ there is no pretence that you're trying to control the flow or the ultimate effect. Rather, you are creating *a more effective application or initiation* during the session. And, in this, the greatest tool, the primary mechanism in the technique is the mind.

In his book, *Psycho-Cybernetics*, Maxwell Maltz said, "*The new science of Cybernetics has furnished us with convincing proof that the so called "sub-conscious mind" is not a "mind" at all but a mechanism – a goal striving "servo-mechanism" consisting of the brain and the nervous system, which is used by, and directed by, the mind.*"

No, this isn't "positive thinking" or "affirmation", "visualization" or "manifestation". Conscious thought plays only a small part although no less important. What I am talking about here is **intent**: an essential element in the process. This is, as it is with the frequencies we deal with, very simple and clear. It's not to be altered through practices brought about by fear or greed or ego. I dare say that is the most difficult part of this entire process; *to not interfere with it.*

This of course brings us back to fear, and whether or not

you allow fear to rule you.

When I first recognized these frequencies within me, there was a true element of the chaotic about me. Like a tap that hadn't been screwed together properly, there were leaks and a total lack of directive flow whenever I turned the energy on. I put the focus on my hands, as I was taught to do, but I'm sure if you were able to see the energy you would have seen little jets sprouting all about, and off, me, as I implemented a session.

Extraordinarily during session, you can pick up the energy around the room, not just off the patient, and have the patient respond. Perhaps that is why. Perhaps we're all leaky taps. People are spouting energy all about the place. *How* leaky you are is determined by how old you are, and how much crap you've been through! It could explain why children flow so well, and why you spend the initial session with some older clients, or someone that has been chronically ill, almost "injecting" energy into them to encourage that system to flow. Perhaps we rust out as we get older! Considering recent findings into cellular membrane and structure, and the communication between those cells, the term "rust" isn't that far-fetched.

One of the harder concepts for our course participants to grasp is that a huge percentage of the frequencies can come from the eyes. I would venture to say the majority do. When I was originally shown this, it didn't make any sense as I watched twenty people stare at a spot where they considered a chakra to be, while another twenty lay on the tables, receiving these stares and waiting for something miraculous to happen. Sadly, for the most part not much did.

However, I realized when I turned my own eyes to the task, I effectively "turned them on". There were no conscious questions or directive, merely recognition that it was occurring, *intent*, and it did. I distinctly felt it, something akin to a huge "wave" of energy crash through my pupils and continue to flow, and you can feel it continuing to flow as the body before me responded. The person on the table was immediately responsive, with greater physical registers than ever.

I referred to the subconscious mind as a "servo-mechanism", through which you could "switch" the frequencies on as needed. But to take one step back and blatantly state the obvious, we access that mechanism through conscious thought.

Peggy Phoenix Dubro, originator of the EMF Balancing Technique™ and author of *Elegant Empowerment*, states, "*It is the wilful cooperation of Conscious Spiritual elements that engineer the required energetic patterns to create change and transformation at our physical levels.*"

There has to be a starting point in this process. And for us, the most accessible and precise starting point is our own mind set, our own balanced accurate thought. You can choose to shape your thoughts so that they actually create energy. This is how you create your own reality. You can use your internal spiritual feeling and that true heartfelt knowledge to propel you into situations that you deserve and that you have planned for. How?

Intent. The single decision to "do". Intent is the key element in instigating the process from conscious thought to action, and right through to spiritual endeavour. That primary intent reaches to the sub conscious level where an intuitive knowledge resides, an intuitive knowledge that I honestly believe every human alive possesses. There is wisdom at a cellular level that understands this spiritual knowledge, and reacquaints itself with the task at hand.

In your effective application of frequency, conscious intent is primary. It is no less important for the client. Your client/patient's intent is also crucial. This is also why you cannot own responsibility for another person's healing or their lack of healing. Remembering that it is only *your* thought over which you have control, you cannot take ownership or responsibility, if, in their heart, your patient has no intent of healing.

I honestly know it to be true, that there is *always* a healing. It is not always what the person on the table would have chosen, but there is always a healing. It isn't always what I would choose, but then, I go in knowing that. I still get my hopes up. And there are times, in my human-ness when I am as disappointed as the client. Healing is not always what you might anticipate…

Healing encompasses many things; there is healing of the soul, of relationships, and of the body. Sometimes it is to quieten those inner voices, or rest that weary heart, or indeed to heal that body. Someone walks in with a broken hand, and walks out healed. Someone else walks in with chronic disease and walks out with it still, but also with knowledge of the lesson that disease brings with it. Spirit holds just for you a carefully drafted plan.

People "own" this, because they already knew it. Within the cell, within the matrix of unknown gaps, there is memory. Bizarre as the experience can be on the table they absolutely know it wasn't a dream or a hallucination. People smelled it, tasted it, heard it, felt that touch. They know it, in their heart, to be true.

Your consciousness is the actual reality. The physical is only temporary. Your cellular structure, although a sacred vessel in itself, is only a place where the Spirit of your consciousness resides, and you can take that spirit anywhere you want. Wherever your thoughts are, your reality is.

The downfall of the human mind is often rooted in emotion. Emotion also makes facilitating this so much harder. When emotion is ruling you, you'll find the flow of these frequencies is lessened, the process more unnatural which, of course, creates a catch 22 effect. You start to doubt yourself and more emotion kicks in and around it, goes. Nothing will stop you on your enlightened journey faster than the belief that you don't deserve it.

Make the decision right now to not let your thoughts venture there. You do deserve this. This gift always was and is for you. This is your time, right now, and it is the right time. If you don't believe it, know that I do, and you can believe me instead.

More than any other instruction pertaining to these frequencies, instrumental application is the hardest to describe and teach in the written word. In workshops, from the evidence I have seen, I can rely on that intrinsic knowledge, that memory to recognize this when it is felt. I can describe it until I am blue in the face, but as soon as a participant *feels* me turn the frequency up and down, their subconscious remembers and recognizes this ability, and they are able to then do it. They reactivate it in themselves.

There will be a way to hand this to you better in the written word. I'll figure it out, hopefully by the next book! For now, the workshop is the most effective way to teach this.

The Instrumental Body™, is now the title of one of the courses we teach, and it turns out, has morphed itself to be almost entirely focused on the ability to self heal. The course was brought about when I could no longer fit in all the details I wanted to in the time we had in the Healing Facilitation course. The Instrumental Body™ is about enhanced application of the frequency, but even I did not know, until we applied it, how effective it could be as a healer of self.

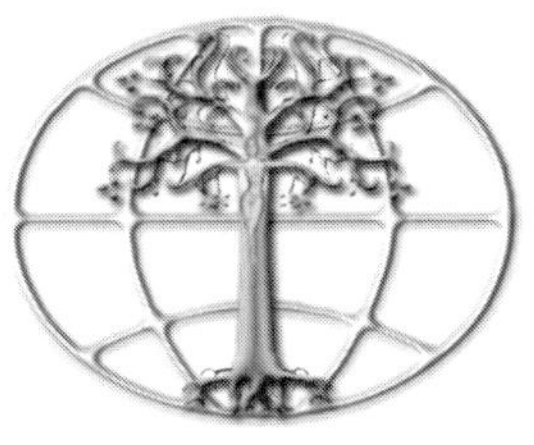

What will you do with this?

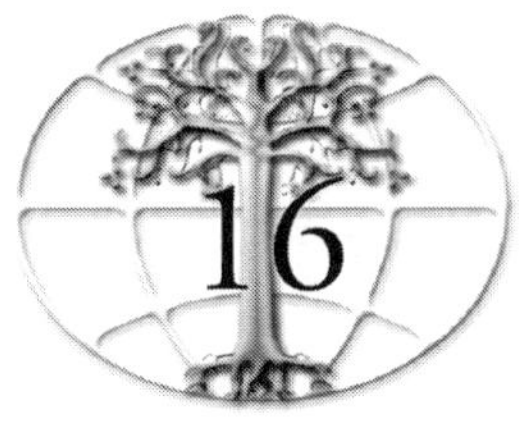

If you can walk, you can dance
If you can talk, you can sing
Traditional Zimbabwe

Enhancement Extras

Let's get back to you and reignite that spark you've found within, because it's time to enhance it further! Let's get back to basics. Rediscover the frequencies as they flow through you. Remember, arms by your sides, wrists back, drop those shoulders… Got it? Can you feel the sensation flowing through that point in your palm; through the pericardium 8?

Now find that little ball of playdough again. If you don't recall the "little ball", go back to the lesson where you were first introduced and go through it again. Go at your own pace. There is no rush. This is your journey. Nobody is testing you or judging you. This is your gift and it can only be beneficial that you familiarize yourself with it in the best way, and at the best pace, for you. Really get to know it. When you're familiar again, "snowball" it, and add a little more "playdough". Feel the size of the ball increase. Feel your own sensory feedback grow.

Your first enhancing exercise…

The ball is rolling

Have you got the ball between your hands? Can you feel it? You will love this one…

It is important in this exercise that you do not close your eyes. Keep your eye on the ball... or at least on your hand.

With your hands still in position with the ball, have a quick feel if it's there with your upper hand. Now take your upper hand away, just comfortably drop it away, leaving the lower hand where it is – palm up.

Looking at the hand left with the ball, you can still *feel* the ball sitting in the palm of your hand, can't you?! Not just in physical presence there, but in something akin to weight.

I know, pretty cool! It gets better…

Keeping your palm facing up and keeping your eyes on the ball, rotate your wrist just gently so that the ball is lightly propelled and rolls around the palm of your hand. Do it exactly the same way that you would if you had a rubber ball in your hand; it's just a slight fluid movement… and you can actually feel the ball rolling about in your hand.

(*author's note; this is so much easier to teach, live, than to write!*)

Again, play with it. Really feel it moving, feel the presence of it slip about the palm of your hand. Roll it in the opposite direction.

Now try it in your other hand. The one you dropped away. No doubt the first hand you tried this in, is the hand you can "feel" more in. For the sake of future reference, we'll call it your "favourite hand".

Rest assured it's quite normal that one hand will feel these frequencies differently from the other. Don't mistake that one hand is weaker than the other, they're just different. There are many theories why this is the case: perhaps one hand is transferring different information to the other, yin and yang, etc. Or perhaps is as simple as biological asymmetry in your physical body, altering flow somehow. It is curious, but ultimately irrelevant, for the frequencies flow through you as they need to.

Ball toss

There are two ways we can do this one, and considering our "ball" familiarity, let's keep going with that first.

You have the sensory ball in the palm of your favourite hand, and again, roll it about a little, familiarize yourself again with the sensation and the presence of its form. Bring your other hand back into the game now. Bring it up in its relaxed anatomical position, and both of your hands are palm up, side by side (like an English cricket outfielder).

Again feel the ball in your hand, roll it a little, then through a natural little flip of your wrist, toss the ball so that it arcs up and over into the upward facing palm of your other hand. And again, it is important that you keep your eyes open, not necessarily on your hands, but open. *Appendix 1, diagram VI.*

Bizarre but true, the feeling of the ball leaving one hand and landing in the other is palpable. Now, roll the ball about in your other hand, where the ball landed, then flip it and toss it back again. Each time the ball lands in your hand, before tossing it again, roll it about in your palm a little, and feel it again.

If your jaw isn't on the ground right now, please stop, take two fingers and check your pulse. This is incredible stuff, isn't it?

This particular exercise is a favourite of mine because within it is the question of how all things are connected and of all things not being of matter, but of energy. For in my own hands this "ball" of frequency holds probably more sensation and substance than an actual rubber ball would. Sometimes physicality seems crude, amid our luminous presence.

I know this exercise, tossing the ball, is a little harder to do, and rest assured not everyone gets it first time. There is another way, in fact my preferred way, of transferring the frequencies between hands. Try this one…

The sands…

Of course, familiarize yourself again first in whatever manner suits you. Know the frequencies as they choose to be sensed in you.

With both hands in the relaxed anatomical position, both palms up, this time in your favourite hand there is a small pile of dry, fine grained, white sand. Look at the hand the sand is in, and feel the substance and sensation of it. Rotate your wrist, slightly, as you did when rolling the ball and you will feel the sand slip and the weight shifting in your palm as it moves about.

Raising the hand with the sand a little higher than your other hand, just as you would with actual sand, tilt your hand and pour the sand into the receptive hand. There's no need to flip one hand over onto the other, the motion is the same as if you had real sand in your hand: you'll feel it slip from one, and the weight and mass transfer to the other. Then tip it back again. *Appendix 1, diagram VII.*

Unlike the ball, this exercise gives you the opportunity to stretch distance a little. Lift the hand with the sand up a little higher and tip the sand from a height. The frequencies getting stronger with distance become even more palpable in their viscous sand-like state. During workshops, as we walk people through this, quickly the sensation develops until participants, instead of feeling the sand land in the receptive hand, feel it falling through it!

The ball is not a ball at all…

Just in case you may have started to pigeon-hole these frequencies, making them fit back into the comfort zone as something linear of mass, or matter or shape…

Go all the way back to the *little* ball. Become familiar

with it again, and then once it is distinctly present, again roll it about in the palm of one hand…found it? With the hand that isn't busy, the hand without the ball let it drop down by your side in its open position, facing forward. Keep moving the ball in your favourite hand, but focus on what you can feel in the hand by your side.

You can feel it, can't you? Things are not always as they seem. One hand isn't sending it to the other, there is no direction, and yet somehow the other hand is experiencing the sensation the first hand is, it is clearly present.

Now, keeping the ball rolling about in your favourite hand, looking at it as you do, focus now on what is happening on the top of your left foot… Try the same again, and focus on the sensation on your forehead.

Every cell knows what every other cell is doing.

It can be difficult to grasp the concept that all things are connected. Perhaps in this it is a little easier, in view of human biology, to accept the cellular "community experience"; each cell has complete knowledge of what is occurring, whether directly related (the hand with the ball) or not. Let's not blow ourselves, or our minds, out of the water just yet… there is more to follow.

These frequencies actually defy the classical definition of "energy", in the fact that with distance they get stronger. How about you test this out?

Familiarize yourself with the frequencies between your hands again, by using your concentrated areas and moving the hands a little larger than the small ball. You want a strong connection, which after the previous exercises won't be a challenge at all.

Play with that connection. Your hands do not have to be one on top of the other: find the position that is comfortable for you. This is your gift, remember?

With one palm facing up and the other above it, start to stretch the connection. Leave the lower hand where it is and start to stretch the other hand upward, maintaining the connection. Every few inches, stop and play with the frequency a little, then stretch it a little further moving your hands a little further apart. If you lose the connection, which can happen when you're learning about this, then drop your hands, shake your shoulders out, and start again.

Generally, people resist this process of stretching the frequencies, instinctively, or perhaps their resistance is conditionally set. If you've worked in a form of energy healing before, you are even more likely to have to fight some conditioned ingrained paradigm. But you will win over it, because if you've worked in energy healing before, you more than most can see the incredible shift these frequencies house.

For the rest of us, we resist because classical physics, the physics we know and the physics that has a solid determined answer, also resists this. The concept of anything energetic becoming stronger with distance, even though we may logically tell ourselves is the case, goes against all we have been taught until recent times. How does it affect us?

Most people get their hands about a foot apart, without prompting, and then stop about there. When I teach this I have to keep pushing, keep encouraging people to *stretch* this, *feel* the difference. In this simple palpable demonstration, we see the quantum base of the frequencies: you can feel an increase in sensation as the distance grows. *It gets stronger with distance.*

This form of healing and the capabilities and discoveries within are unprecedented and its here in our time! And so to you I say, maintain the connection gradually, by the process we mentioned before, and stretch these frequencies until your hands can get no further apart. Go on. I dare you! Because if you are going to be all that you can be, it's going to take a little daring.

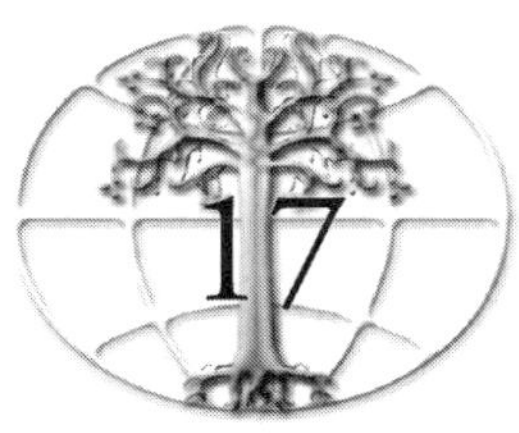

"Not all those that wander are lost."
J. R. R. Tolkien

Working on someone else

Practicing on someone else is a great place to start. Ask someone familiar – a relative, a friend, your partner. The best way to approach them is to put it plainly, "I've just learnt this new *healing thing* (technical term) can I practice on you? It's supposed to be amazing."

This is a great way to start because you've offered your test subject no preconceived ideas or expectations. So everything they tell you they experience will be authentic.

If you can persuade your friend to go the whole hog and get on the table, all the better, because you want to work across the body.

When a client gets on the table, and they're comfortable and settled, I tell them:

"Your task is to 'switch off' and relax. Already you'll notice that your body is relaxing into the table. You'll find that your mind clears and you don't need to think. The whole time you are on the table you will be able to hear me moving about, the birds outside, and the general white noise of life happening as it should. Involuntary physical reactions are normal, and your job is to not let them distract you. Trust me, I've seen a lot, but if you do surprise me, I will let you know.

Throughout the session I won't touch you. The only time I do, is when the session is over. I'll let you know, by touching your shoulder, like so (demo of shoulder touch). If you are worried for any reason, at any stage, just open your eyes."

All of this will become much clearer…

Your client needs to know about the 'switching off' element of the introduction. They shouldn't talk to you during the session (try not to get annoyed when they do, they're just trying to help). Ideally, even though it's someone close to you, you want to distance yourself as much as you can from the familiarity you have with this person. This way you can truly explore these frequencies through an entire body without thinking, "Well, there should be something near his knee. He ruptured that ligament fifteen years ago."

Let's start.

Do you recall how to get your hands into position? We're going to call this "base", so when you need to you can go "back to base". Shake out the shoulders, bring your hands up in their relaxed anatomical position, and have a little play between your own hands, doing whatever little exercise you like best, feeling for the frequencies. If you're nervous or tense at any stage in session, drop your hands away from the body, step back, and shake the old shoulders out and relax. Go "back to base" and then get back into the session.

Discovering the cushion beneath your hands

When you work over or around a body, there is a naturally occurring and quite palpable *gap* between your hands and the body. You may have noticed, during the enhancement exercises, that your hands when transferring these frequencies don't want to be close to one another. The sensation becomes somewhat contaminated if the hands are too close in proximity, by standard physical sensory feedback (standard energy system response, temperature, pressure, etc, quite distinctly different in sensation to frequency response).

It is remarkable just how obvious and easily felt this gap or cushion is. Quite clearly it is the frequencies at work, as once you have discovered this cushion, the physical fatigue from holding your arms or hands in a certain way is non existent. This cushion is a gift in itself. Your hands will glide across the body almost effortlessly, apparently defying gravity as we know it, as these frequencies flow.

You will recognize this cushion with or without a body to work over. However, when charging the environment over which you will work, an actual body to work over makes it all the easier and more obvious again. So if you have a willing friend, do this before the actual session (it will start the flow of frequency for the session anyway).

So go "back to base", getting your hands into a relaxed anatomical position, ready for action. Then, bending at the elbow, bring both hands up to a ninety degree angle in the crook of the elbow. The palms of your hands should be facing the floor, your hands, unchanged in their position. Go on, have a look.

If you have the advantage of working over someone, after raising your forearms and directing the palms to the floor move toward the lower leg area of your client. It's always best to warn the client/friend before you do this. Gently lay your hands on top of the lower leg in front of you, so that your hand naturally curves over the top of the limb. Allow them to take the curvature of the leg, then without changing the shape of your hands lift them off about six inches. Look at your hands. Perfect shape and form, and open; a relaxed anatomical position.

In both situations, with or without a body, we move to 'charge the field', and hence discover your cushion beneath your hands. With your hands where they are, start to slowly move your hands in horizontally elongated ovals, one to two feet in length, and no more than six or seven inches high. This is done on a plane, as if you're wiping a counter top; make three slow ovals. Then stop, lift your hands two or three inches higher and do the same: three slow, elongated ovals. When complete, do it again. Lift two or three inches, then three slow, elongated ovals.

Really *feel* the ovals. Mechanical movement is no asset to you as you're learning this. This is *felt.*

Your three sets of three ovals complete, pause after your last set. Then, again bending at the elbow, raise your forearms, with your hands still in their relaxed position, so that your hands are near your shoulders and your palms are facing forward (the girly "oh my god!" position). Keeping your shoulders and the muscles relaxed and bending at the elbow, do not look at your arms as they move, and gently drop your forearms down until they stop where *they* want to. *Appendix 1, diagram VIII.*

You'll find that at a certain point, as your forearms are dropping, you'll feel a pressure beneath your hands, where your lower arm in its entirety becomes buoyant and floats on a cushion of frequency. Palpable buoyancy in that the charged field that you just created supports the physiological weight. Incredible but true.

Your hands are buoyed upon a distinct charged area that leaves the process of holding your arms in this position almost effortless. A cushion of charge.

This cushion beneath your hands is a primary tool, a given in this gift, that ensures an ease in the facilitation process. Automatically, due to the presence of this cushion, your hands will glide across a body an appropriate distance from the actual flesh, so that the frequency feedback is paramount. You're able to facilitate a session without giving thought to accidentally knocking or hitting the body. Your hands will slip across the body finding what they need to, gliding with unnatural but comfortable ease.

For most people this cushion exists around waist height, a little above or below. If you're having trouble finding it, I have to ask…Are you trying too hard? Are you controlling movement muscularly? Shake out your shoulders, take deep breaths in and out, raise your hands to your shoulders and *relax* and let them drop forward.

If you are privileged to have a test subject beneath your hands, try this out, though it is not essential. You can do this without a body beneath your hands. You're charging a field, not a body. Go through the exercise again, away from a body, of dropping your hands onto your charged cushion. You can actually feel its presence, can't you? Like a buoy or a shelf under your hands.

Working over a body

In order to initially trigger the body and awaken the recognition within it, working around the head is a great place to start. Position yourself standing above the head of your subject, off the end of the treatment table.

In the beginning, approach with one hand only at the temple area on the head of your client. Your initial approach toward the body is similar to the drop in process of finding that charged cushion. With your elbow bent and your hand in a relaxed position, drop just one hand down from your shoulder, bending through the elbow so that the palm of your hand moves across the temple of your subject's head, about six or eight inches away from the temple itself. The palm of the hand is facing the midline of the body you're working on.

Slowly, and I mean *slowly* because you are trying to *find* this energy as it flows through this body, move your hand across the temple area. The palm of your hand should be perpendicular to the direction of the frequency, so the palm of your hand should be facing the temple. Slowly move your hand in a circular motion, finding that sensation in your hand that tells you the connection with the frequencies. You've felt this in your hands before: you know the appropriate sensation.

At the outset, the physical responses make themselves obvious. Even if your subject is sitting in a chair at the kitchen table, these registers are quite clear. The eyes start their fluttering, or oscillating, and your subject will feel it too (this is that moment when they usually start chatting to you about it). If you think it's exciting when you find these frequencies within you, wait until you see them in action on someone else, because you are there assisting them!

Now drop your other hand in too. Bring it down slowly across the other temple, feeling for it.

Your hands remain independent of one another. As in ordinary life, your hands do not and should not move together. There is no synchronized hand movement in this. If you find yourself impersonating the little red engine, doing little synchronized circles on either side of your subjects head (chugging noises are optional) go back to your base…step away from the body, drop your hands, shake out the shoulders, bring your hands up…and start again. Get back into it.

When you work across a body there are certain areas that are clearly felt and make themselves known. Not so coincidentally, they are very similar to known and recognized chakras in the human body.

As you are starting to work about the head, the temples, the crown area of the head (off the top) and of course the third eye area (mid lower forehead) there will usually be a definitive sensory response as the frequencies flow abundantly; likewise other chakra areas such as mid-throat, over the heart area, etc. Gently travel down the midline of the body, and you are sure to feel a response along the way. Play with it as you go. Feel it. Stretch it out and watch as the body embraces and responds to it.

As you work upon a body, moving over it, the frequency calls you to certain spots, certain areas on the body where you will feel more pressure, or pull, energy or general sensation. This is usually around an injury site, such as an injured knee, or fractured bone, or a specific area requiring attention, such as a cancerous tumour. And it's because these areas require balance that you are called to them.

In the same manner, this energy will let you know when to move on from that attention-seeking spot. The frequency will diminish in its sensation to the point of feeling much the same as the rest of the body. An area of unbalance directs you to work over it, then as the frequency is applied and allowed to flow, the effected area returns to a state of balance, and now feels much the same in flow as the rest of the body. The effected area resumes the unique consistent "hum", pertinent to that body. To you, the facilitator, it can feel simply as if you have become bored with that spot and so it's time to move on across the body. These frequencies will talk to you through your body even to the point of letting you know when the session is complete.

Physical Response

There are physical registers that come into play during a session, almost always. Again I have to stress that each client and each session is unique and distinct. Fortunately most people will show you they are actively in session through some physical registers at the primary level. If I were to put a figure on it, from my own experience, eighty-five percent of clients will demonstrate these registers, at a minimum.

And thank goodness, because human self esteem can be a fickle thing! If we, facilitating the session, are not seeing some sort of response, our first reaction is, "Well, obviously, *I* can't do it. Everyone else has the ability to do this, just not me." Rather than dealing with ego, here lies the need to combat the faltering of self esteem within. Self esteem and the challenges in maintenance is what we were referring to when we discussed quieting the "static" in your own mind. For it is when the seeds of doubt enter the self esteem and it takes a battering, that static creeps in.

Primary registers

The eyes

The first register you experience, or as a facilitator will witness on the table, is eye flickering. This is the most common of the primary level of registers that you see. The eyelids flutter, lower and upper, like a rapid partial blink. This fluttering can be slight, where the eyelashes appear to tremor, or be so strong that the eyelids themselves cannot stay closed. This fluttering can go throughout the entire session, or as the client goes deeper into the session will slow and cease as the eyes move into a secondary level response: a pattern of oscillation with the eyeball moving rhythmically and measured, side to side, beneath the eyelid. You'll find you won't be guessing if these registers are occurring or not. They are quite plainly visible.

Breathing

Still within the realm of primary registers, you may notice the clients breathing alters. When on the table, for the most part, this change in breathing goes unnoticed. Initially it kind of relaxes, becoming a little lighter, shallower and rhythmic. A slight shudder may start in the diaphragm. From our side it appears that the diaphragm is running up and down a little staircase, with each inhale and exhale.

As the client goes further into session, their breathing can alter quite dramatically, even to the point of apparently not breathing at all, as you may recall from Stuart's session. The theory behind a client not breathing at all is that wherever they are, they are at the point, or at such a level, that they don't need to breathe. Not at this end anyway.

The first few times I saw this, it was hard not to panic. I would put my ear close to the client's chest, desperate to hear the comforting rush of air through the lungs, but nothing. I would watch the client closely for any signs of oxygen deficiency, watching for the first inclination of discoloration around the lips. Two, then three minutes, not so much as a hint of blue was showing. In the client's debriefing after the session, some would remember not breathing, and recall thinking, apparently just in passing, 'Oh, I'm not breathing' but chose to do nothing about it. More often than not what made them realize it was that first intake of air when they did resume breathing. I learned to trust this.

At the session's end, when I embrace the clients shoulder and welcome them back, I await their first deep inhalation before I step away from them. That drinking in of air is akin to a coming back to awareness for them.

Swallowing

Usually quite early in the session, clients will swallow loudly and awkwardly. If they are having trouble letting go, this register makes them more self conscious again. On the table this feels awkward and a little uncomfortable simply because you have to think about an action that is usually involuntary. It's a register that is common, usually early in the session, and most times will only last for a swallow or two.

Head movement

Another common register you're likely to see is movement of the head. The side to side rolling of the head, sometimes only slight, sometimes quite pronounced is the movement you see most often. The head tilting back or nodding, are likely to be seen too.

Fine motor

Fine motor movements such as fingers tapping, or flicking, or hand flexion, are again normal (whatever that is!). Wrists will tilt in a variety of directions, hands will actually lift up and away from the body and the table, and usually, not coincidentally, in a static relaxed anatomical position. All this, too, is common. Toes move too – a twitch here, a flexed toe there. Feet will plantar and dorsa flex, rotate, etc.

Gross motor

Nearly every client experiences gross motor twitches and movements at some level or another. Muscles through their back or mid section twitch and flex. Legs and arms move, lifting, bending, rotating, and vibrating. Sometimes, most times, they simply experience effectively a twitch. I have to generalize here because the scope for variation in this type of movement is infinite.

Facial

All the muscles in the body, operating through the responsive electrical system as muscles do, have the potential to respond to these frequencies. And all have, in one person or another. This being the case, the facial response and the muscular complexity that makes up the face, warrants a paragraph all its own.

All clients demonstrate some level of response through the expressions upon their face. The muscle twitches through the face, being such a complex myriad of muscle structure, are quite amazing to watch. Every possible expression of emotion visibly romps across the client's face. Apparently my own face goes berserk when I'm on the table, although I can honestly tell you I don't once recall actually feeling it do so. But too many have confirmed it.

Children in particular go to the extreme: a huge smile is triggered, then in a split second the deepest of frowns comes in, then back to another, but equally huge, smile, then a grimace, a frown, a grimace, a sneer, a smirk… and the dance continues. Kids often get the giggles, and vocalize too. So the facial response in a child is an experience in itself.

Emotions

At this point, recognizing the experience people have on the table and respecting that experience, you should be prepared for any emotional response the client may demonstrate whilst in session. More often than not, the client is completely unaware that they are doing anything audible or even physical whilst on the table during the session.

Do be prepared for the emotional response at the close of the session too. Keep the tissues in supply, and understand that such a transition for any individual is bound to bring about at least a little emotional upheaval.

Tears

During session people often have tears forming in their eyes, if they don't actually start crying. Crying entails anything from unaccounted tears quietly coursing down their face, to the all involved sobbing. It's hard to say whether this is a rudimentary physical response or if it's a far deeper response beyond conscious recognition, not unlike the "easing" of the heart. Perhaps it's simply *relief.* These days everyone could use a little of that. Regardless, you will see this in most clients. So as I mentioned, keep a box of tissues handy for the salvaging of make up, and the immediate reduction in masculine embarrassment ("It *is* dusty in here, sir. You must have got a little in your eye.")

When I say I've seen an awful lot in these sessions, I'm not joking. I've had clients curling up in the foetal position and sucking their thumb. People have screamed or wailed and cried as if their heart was breaking, laugh uncontrollably (and complained of abdominal muscle soreness the next day), giggle like little girls, and bluster like politicians.

I've watched as bodies have shuddered and convulsed with muscle contractions. Bodies have been writhing and squirming. People suddenly sit up, straight up without any assistance, then slowly melt back down to lying on the table. Limbs seem to explore the space around them in a slow, constant movement. A straight leg lifts off the table and starts to rotate, or a straight arm extends away from the body unsupported, and utterly defying gravity, holds the posture for thirty or so minutes.

During his Axial Initiation™ a man arched up off the table so that only the back of his head and his heels were touching the table. I mean the physics of holding this posture alone are pretty incredible. Gymnasts around the world would be impressed.

The majority of people you'll work on won't be so dramatic in response or registers (hopefully). As I mentioned earlier I've found it an asset to diminish the distracting physical response wherever I can. On the other hand, if they are physically dramatic you can email me and know you have a comrade in healing. It's always good to have an understanding friend.

Some of the less common and yet not unlikely registers you may experience, or under another title, "some of the weird stuff I've seen", may include:

Hair movement

You know when you put a helium balloon near your hair and you get that very stylish static electricity look as your hair clings to the balloon? Yes, hair does this with my hands. As I work around the head, the hair moves and follows my hands. I know you're visualizing some extreme sci-fi image right now, but it's more subtle than that. Any relatives present in the room love it, and it's a topic that always comes up after the session. It says something for the electromagnetic presence within these frequencies, doesn't it?

Little unborn wonders

I've been fortunate enough to work on quite a lot of babies that were still in-utero, one of my favourite sessions, really. The little babies chase your hands around if you're near the body, or when you're moving around the table they follow you whilst still in the womb. Very sweet. Mothers, who have experienced no obvious movement during the pregnancy, suddenly have a lot of movement. The babies just love it!

There have been dramatic results from these sessions for the babies too. When I receive a call requesting I work with an unborn child that has been diagnosed with challenges, they are usually calling me to request I meet them at the hospital when the child is born. I'm not opposed to doing just that, even though it invariably means I enter the neonatal intensive care unit to work on them (not a place of fond memory for me).

From the very first enquiry of this kind, it seemed far

more logical to me to work with the child while it remained in-utero. In this way it could take advantage of the mother's established physiological system, and of course the incredible life support of the placenta. The alternative was waiting until the child is born, with its undeveloped immune system, and basic struggle to adapt to life as a physical human…a newborn has enough to adjust to. At least in-utero the battle is shared. And there have been some truly miraculous changes in these tiny warriors.

Channelling on the table

I have to tell you this is not something I would have ever anticipated, or welcomed if I had known it was coming. The first time I had someone channel on the table was during an Axial Initiation™ with a woman called Cherie. At first, during the first session, I thought I must have misheard a tummy rumble or something, and then I saw this lady's mouth moving. Initially it was moving silently, but as I continued through the process, it turned into a whisper. I couldn't hear what she was saying, no matter how hard I tried. The pounding of my own heart obliterated any hope of hearing it, really. I pride myself on finishing the session without freaking out and running away quickly.

I'm an Anatomical Physiologist. My clients didn't channel! I had heard of this before, but it was not meant to happen to me. Freaky! Images of *The Exorcist* were flashing through my mind.

As we were debriefing afterwards, she told me all about her session, what she saw, who she spoke to, and when I thought she had finished, I looked up and said, "Anything else?"

Too quickly she said, "No!"

The second session, the channelling was loud and clear almost the instant I started the procedure. Her voice changed

(Cherie had a strong Pakistan accent), in intonation and articulation, but not in pitch. There was no screeching or strangely adaptive vocals like those some associates had mentioned. It was Cherie's voice, but there was no doubt that this was not Cherie talking.

As we already know, my etiquette when it comes to interacting with channelling entities needs work. Apparently I'm not appropriately silent in my reverence. Maybe it's the sceptic in me, but I wanted to know what this particular entity was up to. Around this time, being fairly new to it all, I had been hearing about the evil spooks and negative energies that were allegedly trying to attack me (I'd only recently managed to peel my fingers away from the nape of my neck where they were likely to assault me). I had to wonder if this was one of them. So I started asking questions. Oddly, I didn't ask *who* it was.

The voice started telling me that this work had to be "enhanced", that there was "more to follow" and that I must "go forward" (again). Bossy! Then it spoke of balance, both for the client and for me (please note I am holding nothing back from you. You've heard all that I have.) I asked questions, even argued a little, and the conversation went on for about 25 minutes. Throughout the rest of the session Cherie displayed "normal" registers. When I touched her shoulder, she nearly head-butted me, she sat up so fast! Her eyes were huge. However, she remained silent.

I asked, "Can you speak?"

A little hope entered the expression on her face, "Did I speak at all during the session?"

"Quite a lot actually..."

"It wasn't me! I don't know what happened! It wasn't me, Melissa! I'd never speak to you like that! I'd never boss you around like that!" I told you, he was bossy.

Like my friend Helen, Cherie had felt the need to speak and had done everything she could not to. Unlike Helen,

Cherie heard it all, both the entity and my conversations, and had wondered who I was talking to.

From the client's perspective, this can be pretty disturbing. I'm not going to pretend to know much about channelling. Should you see someone do this, try to put on your poker face and act like it's normal. In regard to appropriate channelling etiquette; I have no real answers for you, save this:

- Trust your gut. You do know if this entity channelling through is someone genuine or not, trust your intu ition. Believe it or not, people will pretend!

- Always hold such an experience in the highest esteem, and treat it with the utmost respect.

- Above all, be grateful for it. After all, it was a gift in lesson, plainly handed to you.

- Take notes. I do.

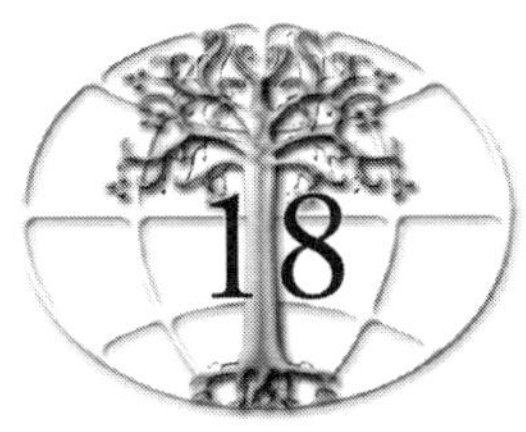

"Keep me away from the wisdom that does not cry,
the philosophy that does not laugh
and the greatness that does not bow before children."
Kahlil Gibran

Ritualistic Endeavour

M***editation***

You're deep enough into the book now, to know me fairly well. I'm going to get a little blunter.

Can you even imagine how many of the people that come to me, see what I do and offer me advice? Rest assured I always listen. After all I am still learning, and this experiential education continues. I don't however, always take this advice on. Just as I offered to you in the introduction: I take what I need, discard what I don't, and sincerely hope I have enough wisdom to know the difference.

Early on, when I was seeing clients, the advice ran thick and fast:

Giving orders: "Protect yourself Melissa! You're taking all their disease on, and you won't last!"

Giving gifts: "I brought this for you to – put in your window/ wear over your heart/ wash your hands in/ close off your heart chakra/ the list is long and very generous."

Conclusions: "You're possessed. That's why this is happening. You're possessed."

Or, "You see? You've betrayed the Lord, and now your hands are on fire." *On fire?*

Personal attacks: "You're not an angel, you know!" Not in this lifetime, anyway.

People from all walks of life, all faiths, all socio-economic mixes, all educations, including the extreme, right brain, new age element, will come in the door. Unsolicited advice is a given, and in some regards, a blessing. Wisdom comes clothed in the strangest garments.

Within a period of one week several people had told me I wasn't meditating enough. *Meditating. Hmmm...* Now it was no coincidence (for there are no coincidences) that a number had mentioned this all in a small space in time, so I considered it. I admit I was not meditating much at all.

When the term 'meditation' is bandied about, I know I tend to think of it as a ritualistic procedure for the purpose of trying to communicate with God. And in this it places us in a position of ritualistic worship, of subservience, or at least it implies that we are in a lesser position and of a lower significance. Now bear in mind this is merely my own interpretation and there is little doubt my upbringing played a part in this mind set.

So I tried to schedule a little extra meditation between the client appointments, breast feeding my youngest daughter, my son's physical therapy, feeding the family, doing the laundry, and running the business. It wasn't fitting in terribly well. I would sit down and ritualistically go through the motions to be ready to meditate, close my eyes and...fall asleep. Not intentionally.

This was also happening if I tried to do a self healing. I

would get comfortable, switch the frequencies on and promptly nod off. You can sleep through a session, and it doesn't mean the frequencies aren't working, it just means you have no conscious connection with it. You miss the experience.

Regardless, the meditation thing wasn't happening. So I became strict in the ritual and process of meditation, disciplining myself. And in the nanoseconds of spare time I had to do this, I found sleep came just as readily.

Discussing this with a friend, she laughed and said, "Mel, what are you doing? Every time you're in session you meditate! How else could you know what you know, or understand what you do?" What a relief!

Meditating without ritual. Actually, even less ritual than no ritual. All it seemed to take is an environment in which the mind could know quiet. I can be hanging the washing out, or sitting in the kid's bedroom as they go to sleep, or in a quiet moment on my own, and the communication is rich and strong and comforting. The answers I seek and the communication I know is clear and prompt.

Even in a noisy or busy environment if my mind can disconnect from the activity it can know quiet. My favourite "meditation" is when I go for a run. My time (exhausted mothers the world over can hear the bliss in the words as I write that!) Another is watching a favourite movie that I've seen before. Simply spending some time in my own company.

Deepak Chopra said of this, "*Spirit whispers to us through the gap between our thoughts and the slightest sensation in our body. This is why spending some time in the silence is so important. When we think of healing as the return of the memory of wholeness and wholeness as body, mind, spirit and environment, we begin to understand why we must learn to quiet our minds.*"

In this process of meditation that I now know, I've come to understand meditation is instrumental in that it is a process where we gain control over the mind, and direct it. Through meditation you can actually alter your thought patterns, breaking out of thought habits instilled throughout a lifetime, and embrace new ones. Like all things evolving right now, in this you cannot deny the spiritual element, but ascension into the "spirit world" is no longer the directive, or goal, in meditation. In itself this isn't ascension, but it is, like the mind itself, no less a significant phase in the process. Instead of reaching out to the external higher source, we need to have the courage to use this tool to look within. After all, that spark of divinity is within, and hence so is God.

Ritual has not been without its place. However no longer is such discipline and stricture required nor is appropriate in this today's evolutionary environment.

The energy on the planet has changed. Ancient frequencies, these frequencies, have shown themselves now and are bringing about healing unprecedented in our time. The biology of the human being, and of any living organism, can respond in a manner previously unknown to us.

Evolution is not mutually exclusive to the human. The vibratory resonance upon the planet has elevated. Nobody is a lesser healer; no modality is "outdated". But it does have to be considered that rituals once placed or designed in an environment that no longer exists, must also change and evolve. You cannot go forward whilst clinging to the past.

The main thing is to keep the main thing, the main thing.

Interference

This process of healing is non-invasive and "hands off". It requires no nudity, no prayer, no crossing of oneself, no salts, and no burning of sage. It requires no protection, guards at the door, chastity belts or *ohms*. You need not remove jewellery, strip yourself of leather, subject your wardrobe devoid of red and black, and please feel free to not contort yourself into any lithe positions. In the event of experiencing nausea, please lean over the side of the table and aim for your own shoes. (Just kidding!)

This gift is, as it is with the frequencies we deal with, very simple and clear. It's not, again like the information, to be altered through practices brought about by fear or greed or ego. No, not even your favourite crystal. I dare say that is the most difficult part of this entire process; *to **not** interfere with it.*

This of course brings us back to fear, and whether or not you allow fear to rule you.

In this the most natural of gifts all interference, including trying too hard, is just that…interference. Any prior blessing, or preliminary processes of any sort, ultimately is hindering the real process for you and the client. Any rituals you might care to put in place prior or during session only open the door to self doubt, both for you and your client. This is not where you want to start.

Someone will ask me what I do for a living and within minutes, rather than languish over explanations, I find myself initiating their hand so they can feel it themselves. I quickly put their hands into a relaxed anatomical position, and then, 'zap'. Soon after they've gathered themselves from the initial wonder of it, they say, "My god, you're not even *trying*!" or something similar. They're right, I'm not.

There is no squinting of eyes in effort as I magically draw this through, I don't spit out a quick Hail Mary before I put my hands near them, and I don't warm up, breathe it through, brace myself or wave my hands about their head to clear away the last of the dust bunnies from their aura. For two reasons: I cannot be bothered, and more importantly, I *do not need to*!

My experience has been that such preliminaries, with the exception of prayer, are far more about self importance, or at least the attempt to appear more important. And with regard to appearances, let's face it, a huge amount of modalities can look like you're waving about a couple of dead fish. I imagine, as most eyes *learn* to see these frequencies, that at first glance I probably look similar when I'm demonstrating! God forbid! In fact in the effortless flow of these frequencies, it probably looks like I'm not doing anything at all other than waving my hands about artistically, except for the feedback of the astonished expression of the person that I am working on.

These frequencies just flow. If you cannot feel them, chances are you are trying too hard. If you cannot see them yet, don't pretend to, and know that you probably will down the track. I can see them visually, but I don't need to. Another comment when I am activating a hand is that I'm not even looking while I do it. These frequencies are based on light and information, and somehow I don't need to look, I just *know* where the hand is, what my hands are doing and how the frequencies are flowing.

As far as combining modalities or professional method with this, you've probably gathered that I am not averse to it. This is to enhance your gift, not dictate it. For your own sake, don't call it something it isn't, or misrepresent yourself through it. You won't fool the frequencies, the flow will diminish, and people are far more astute than you think, so you probably won't fool them either.

Keep it simple, honest, and keep it true to you. Study it, learn from it and enhance where you can. Why interfere with a gift that is so genuine?

Rituals (Fear disguised)

On your enlightened journey nothing will stop you faster than the belief that you don't deserve it.

In the process of transferring or using these frequencies, being emotional is a great hindrance. If you're stressed, depressed, angry, despairing or caught in a web of your own emotional making, the flow of these frequencies will dissipate. This list includes fear. Being emotional slows it down, and slows you down. It affects the flow.

Some healers will tell you that rituals offend, and somehow intrude upon the healing process and they should be utterly thrown out. These same healers will probably tell you that the only healing method or modality is *their* method, and you can only do it with their permission (we'll discuss integrity later). Ritual process has always had its place in the most sacred places, and to assume *all* have been inappropriate or pointless would be simply egotistical.

I'm not highly educated about crystals and their properties. I have received many as gifts, and I like them, but as to their individual innate power, as I said at this stage I remain somewhat ignorant. What I believe to be true, however, is that as long as you ***believe*** that an amethyst will bring calm, moldavite will bring communication, or rose quartz love, just the belief in itself will enable the crystal to do exactly that; as long as you ***believe*** it.

Even if a crystal is only a physical embodiment of a positive affirmation then it remains, still, powerful. While I know far less than many, when it comes to crystals I do know enough of their history, their evolution and their make up to know that they *do* hold incredible power all their own. So imagine the potential if that is put alongside your own belief!

Belief in these frequencies is easy. Before your very eyes you can see a body responding. Within your own body you can palpably feel the sensation. Between your hands you can roll a small ball, present and formed. Confirmation of this healing gift is readily yours. Believing in you is where the challenge truly lies. My advice on this is simple…

Believe in what *you* know to be true in *your* heart.

The majority of rituals have usually been brought about by fear: in healing, usually this is the fear of the uncontrollable and unknown, and in more recent times, fear of litigation.

Some ritual processes are exquisitely beautiful, not to mention self assuring. There are some rituals that do have their place, and to disregard them is, as I said, is a decision based in ego. I said before that operating emotionally does you no favours as a facilitator, and fear, of course, is a base emotion.

Some rituals are simply inappropriate in current times. Fear-based protective ritual only enhances fear itself. Placing guards at the door, smudging the entryway with sage, counting and combining the belief patterns of multiple incense sticks or essences, wearing amulets or even garlic are no asset to you. These and many, many others are considered *protective rituals*, but such fear based protection is, in this, *restrictive.*

The founder of *The Reconnection*, Eric Pearl, has written, "*Being a healer means letting go of the unnecessary stuff that may or may not have served you at some stage, and definitely serves you no longer, except to keep you in a state of attachment. Don't cling. Attachment equals need, which equals fear.*"

Great spiritual teachers and leaders have taught me that nobody, not even the spiritual can harm me, *unless I invite it.* I assure you that while this is stated simply, it is not naiveté.

If someone, spiritual or otherwise, is in your space and makes you uneasy, and every nerve is on edge, you can plainly tell them to get out. And they will. You are far more powerful than you know. Take my word for it. You are actually a piece of God walking the planet in lesson for the sake of a grander purpose. In this newly recognized knowledge, you are now part of the greater plan, with purpose and responsibility.

Should some small ritual, a ritual based on *self* and not on *protection*, create peace in your heart where there was no peace, then by all means… Truly, to be an effective healer, you must be balanced. Your mindset, the thoughts and patterns that dwell within, must also be balanced. If you're nervous, afraid, self conscious and you have ritual that can ease this "static", then I say use it. It can only increase your ability to be vehicle to these frequencies.

Sometimes, just before a session, I take a deep breath and kind of shake out my shoulders. Some tennis players also do this just before they serve. If it's a long day, I'm tired or feeling the stress a little, it's a habit that relaxes the upper body, and convinces my weary body that it can cut a few more laps around the room. Some would call it a ritual!

Please, do not take this out of context! Fear based protective ritual only enhances fear itself. Don't even open the door to it. Holding onto these rituals is denying yourself growth. This is your time, and your time is **now**. Please, don't waste your energies on someone else's paradigm. Don't let fear rule you.

Remind yourself: Darkness cannot exist where there is light. When you walk into a dark room, and switch on the light, does any of the darkness remain? No. In this, as in all things, knowledge is light. The combination of truth, knowledge and wisdom is a truly powerful balance. Where there is knowledge, darkness cannot exist.

Carry your own lantern and you need not fear the dark.

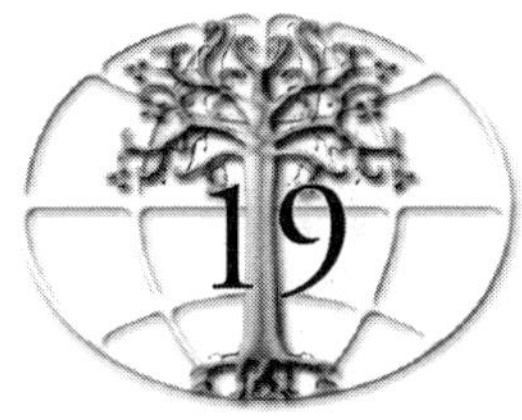

"It is the way of heaven to show no favouritism.
It is forever on the side of the good man.'
The Tao Te Ching, by Lao Tzu

Integrity

Operate from integrity. Always. Ensure that all decisions you make, for yourself first and foremost, stem from what you know to be right.

We are conscious, intelligent human beings. We know what the right thing to do is, and what isn't. Great men have risked life and lost lives, defying a state they were once loyal to, in order to do the right thing. Our task, in a far safer society, is much simpler.

A wise friend and I were discussing the appalling state of the ethics in a business we were both associated with. This particular business was starting to be seen as a bit of a joke, despite the fact that the work they were doing was great. I was commenting on how they had brought it upon themselves, it had been bound to happen, due to their abhorrent business ethics.

My learned friend intoned, "There is no such thing as 'business ethics', Mel. You either have ethics, or you don't. " This is why he is a *wise* friend of mine.

Ethics exist in life, not in circumstance. Integrity without knowledge behind it is fairly weak. But knowledge without integrity is dangerous and often heinous.

I'm told it's an element of being an Indigo, but I can identify a lie long before it's left anyone's lips. And, in my refusal to acknowledge those grey areas, I see a spoken lie, an unspoken truth, and a conscious deception all in the same genre: dishonesty. Early on I decided I needed a plan to deal with people who felt the need to behave like this. I know others came up with variations of this, but my own three-strikes-and-you're-out rule is simple:

The first time someone does you wrong, it could be an accident.

The second time, it's a mistake.

The third time, it's deliberate. You're out.

Not out of my life, or my heart, but never to be trusted.

Prior to this healing gift showing itself to me, I had been in school, university, business and the military. When I came into this new world, this new environment as a Healing Facilitator, I came upon a whole new community unknown to me until then; the New Age crowd.

When I left the Army and re-entered civilian life, I was struck dumb at just how self-involved and malicious people were in order to achieve their own ends. I cannot speak for other international military establishments, but in the Australian military, honour, integrity and loyalty were paramount. Yes, there are always those that don't abide, but for the most part you could rely on the honour and integrity of those serving next to you. Re-entering civilian life, the opposite seemed true: I was better to assume anyone I dealt with was dishonest.

It seemed to me that everyone was stabbing everyone

they could in the back, if not cutting them off at the knees, for their own gains. The horror of watching this behaviour (which I had always lived amongst), was a brutal experience, from my changed perspective.

The New Age crowd, as I mentioned earlier, was a mix of individuals that I couldn't have anticipated. The beauty of people involved in the new age arena is that they are somewhat more advanced in their journey. Already they have experienced an awakening in order for them to merely be present. Yet in this, and I am speaking generally, they can be more sensitive, more reactive, more interactive on multiple levels, and hence what we know as a human reaction and human insecurities, is amplified. Both the good and bad.

In this crowd, amid these audiences, I have experienced beauty and wisdom unlike any other. Oh, the exquisite experience of learning from those more advanced than us! But also, in this crowd, I have seen more people become obsessive, or fall into extreme emotional patterns, born of fear; envy, greed, jealousy, of course, anger, and more. And I see them lose their way, forget what is important, and get lost in a myriad of their own negativity. It is devastating to watch. To see someone forget that they are in fact a fabulous person, but they themselves don't seem to know that any more. They're too busy devising the next dastardly plan to overturn someone else's successes.

I've had some strange obsessive individuals enter my life since I've been working in healing. Female ones! They dye their hair blonde and get it permed (see picture on back cover), and tell people that they are some of my best friends. They are sweet to my face and venomous when my back is turned. They send in spies, to come and have a session with me, and then fire off email full of ridiculous accusations about what I'm doing to whomever they feel might listen. It's a strange and colourful environment.

A few days after I this gift had found me, I found myself

curious, and habitually working on everything. Trying it out, I guess, would be a better term for it, on everything, from the lettuce in the vegetable garden, to my husband's mangled legs, the kids when they were sleeping, and also when they were awake and active to see the different response on this side of the equation. I would be driving the car and a huge wave would rush through me from head to toe.

From the outset, Tim, our cat, just couldn't stay away from these frequencies. Tim by nature is not a big purrer. He does purr, but he's not a floozy with it. Yet when I worked on Tim, he instantly broke into huge purrs: you know the one that has a note to it. The first time I worked on him, just trying it out, straight away you could actually *feel the purr* in the frequencies. As I stretched them, moving away from Tim, and the frequencies got stronger, so did the purring vibration. (It's so much fun, discovering these frequencies!)

This was also a significant moment in my education for another reason. After that introductory period I had attended in Melbourne, one of the participants from the workshop had set up an internet forum for us all to have a chat about what was going on. I was so excited and I was readily sharing all the incredible stuff that was happening! I mean people were just landing on my doorstep for healing, people that I would never have met in my previous existence! It *was* exciting. It still is!

I can be a little gullible I admit, or perhaps I just don't have enough time to trivialize enough, but a certain hostility had been developing toward me. Honestly, I hadn't meant to sound obnoxious, I was just blown away by what had been awoken in me. After a few days, it took someone else to point out that nearly everyone else's comments on the forum were kind of half enthusiastic "good on you, Melissa." or "I have just done my first healing session on my mother" kind of comments. No one else was saying, "The man that had a stroke can speak again", or "a woman's nerve damage was completely repaired".

When I entered the comment about Tim, my friend, Ayesha, pointed out that some back-stabbing was going on. Not long after her warning, we were invited to a dinner with a small group of participants from that first workshop. As it turned out, it was a gathering of the most threatened and apparently envious. At this dinner it became clear that I had offended them and bruised their egos somewhat. Honestly it was unintentional. During the dinner, a group of three women went to great lengths telling me that I was in dire need of healing and that only they should work on me. I politely declined, saying I felt more complete, and better, than I ever had!

Only days later, when I was at home with my kids, I received a call from one of the women. She said, "Hi! Are you at home right now, because we're all in the car on our way over? We're going to do a healing on you." The three of them would not take no for an answer. Every nerve within me was on edge. Something was really wrong here. I knew their intent was to do damage of some sort. I asked where they were, which was about ten minutes away, and threw the kids in the car and left the house.

One of these women in particular, the one who called, years later still wastes an incredible amount of thought-time despising me. Yes, I don't use this terminology lightly. This poor girl has developed this resentment into an absolute hatred of whatever it is in her head that she calls Melissa Hocking. She looks terrible for it! She seems to be self destructing under the weight of it.

It was Mahatma Gandhi who said, "*If a man tries to give you a gift, and you refuse it, who then owns it?*" This poor woman, who actually has a sweet heart, is self destructing because *she* owns her hatred. I owe this woman gratitude, for she was the loudest and most pronounced lesson about people at this stage.

Are you scared now? Are you wondering if you should you do this work? Rest assured you should! And you will not be harmed by individuals of the nature of those I have mentioned, so long as you are true to yourself. For therein lies the definition of integrity: to first be true to yourself.

The society we live in generally has become "fat". Not obese, but lazy in our responsibilities to ourselves and to others, and comfortable to be there. It can appear that people have lost sight of what is truly important, in the race to supersede their neighbour. Yet it seems to me that compromising integrity was never an option.

Do you remember the Golden Rule? We've all heard it no matter what life or religion we grew up in: To do unto others as you would have them do unto you. This isn't about religion, it's about life.

Do you recall why treating a man respectfully is so important? As you sow you shall reap. Call it as you know it; "what goes around comes around", some call it "karma" (loosely interpreted), "what you put out there, you will get back", or "the law of compensation" (for it goes both ways).

Napoleon Hill, in *Law of Success*, wrote "*Every man takes care that his neighbour does not cheat him. But a day comes when he begins to care that he does not cheat his neighbour. Then all goes well. He has changed his market cart into a chariot of the sun.*"

Respect yourself. Respect others. And own responsibility for yourself, your decisions and your actions. You'll be surprised what peace this brings to your own heart.

Prior to undertaking any mentoring or learning at my hand, or through **melissa hocking healing**, I ask that participants read and sign a basic code of conduct. If they don't sign it, then they don't partake in the course or program. It's actually not what you might be thinking. As yet I have never had to hold anyone to it legally, and actually, that was never the intention. My intent is that they *sign* it.

When they sign it, after reading it, they take ownership of the promise. It is then in *their* mind, *they* own it, and it is a responsibility they can ignore but will not be rid of. I don't need to hold them to that code of conduct, for they hold themselves to it. For some individuals, before the course has even begun, they undergo a huge personal shift just in applying a single signature!

Whatever a person chooses to do with their life and their lot is their business. Just don't expect me, or the professional individuals who associate with me, to back you up if you choose something unethical. If you are going to do it, do it well!

And it pays to remember you cannot escape you.

The esteemed Winston Churchill and a colleague of his were walking together down the street. As they strolled on, a woman, clearly a "lady of the night", passed them by and as she did Mr. Churchill tipped his hat to her. His colleague was scandalized, and said, "*Sir, why would you tip you hat to her? Do you not see who she is?*" Mr. Churchill replied "*I do not tip my hat because of who she is. I tip my hat because of who I am.*"

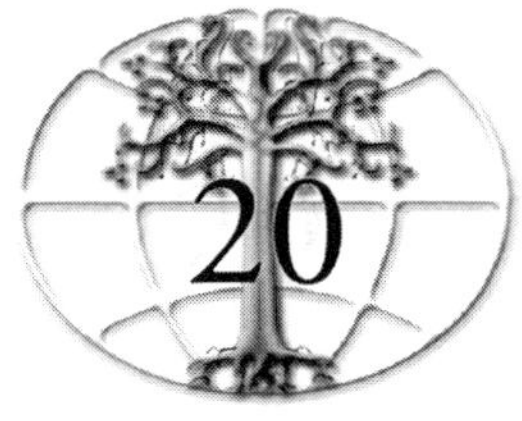

20

"The shortest answer is doing"
English proverb

Environment knows no boundaries

I was working with a friend at his workshops when we were approached by a couple who had flown in from New Zealand with their autistic child seeking a healing session. He offered to do it, and asked if I would help out during the session with this family.

This couple was exhausted, soulfully fatigued, in a way that is almost indescribable. You could feel them, in their utter despair and heart wrenching frustration, the moment you were in their presence. Their seven-year-old son was autistic and was labelled ADHD – attention deficit hyperactivity disorder (you know that undiagnosable-but-readily-diagnosed-and-drugged-anyway disorder? Sorry, I can get a little passionate on this topic).

Before they had arrived I started to restrict the environment – simplifying the hotel room, closing doors, dimming the lighting in the room, decreasing any stressful components for this child. Bear in mind, thanks to my own son, I have spent a lot of time around children with any number of disabilities and any mix of them. My associate is childless and therefore not well versed in the behaviours of children, typical developing or otherwise and so was perplexed by my apparently odd behaviour, as I went about doing this, thinking I was nervous.

When they had arrived, my friend, through lack of experience with kids, was trying to conduct a session "by the book". This was never going to happen. As my friend chased this child over the couch, under the table, around the chair, the boy stopping only to slap away my friend's hands, the tension in the room was increasing exponentially. I don't know how the parents restrained themselves (probably years of practiced patience), because *I* was about to explode. So as my friend raced by in hot pursuit, I reached out and caught his arm, hissing "Stop!"

I went over and took the mother's hand and silently looked into her eyes. Her heart was so tired. And I started to work on her son.

The little boy had landed, sitting down near a corner of the room with his legs hugged into his chest, rocking as he faced the wall. It was so clear he was seeking quiet. I sat down on the floor myself, and, using my eyes, I switched the frequency on and started to immerse him, by charging the area around him. Initially I didn't work directly on him. I let the frequency flow hard, fast and rich, as much as I could allow for it. I felt desperate to bring relief to this family!

They told me later, as I don't recall it, that I apparently started to hum a low repetitive phrase. I know that out of habit and probably for my own comfort, I did start to feel for the boy with my hands. I could see a huge shimmer of frequency, to the point that visually for me the rest of the room was disappearing. The little boy, his back facing me, shuffled his backside back toward me. He had stopped rocking.

This went on for some time, and every now and then his little butt would shuffle a little closer until he was less than a metre away with his back to me. I do recall that he too started to hum a low repetitive phrase. I was moving my hands less than a meter away from him, feeling for any health issues (I mean I may as well, while I was there anyway) and he was not disturbed by it at all.

As I finished the session, I quietly stood up and started to move away, and he turned his head a little. His little cheeks were stained with the tears that had been coursing down them. I turned and embraced that who I could, and who also needed it: his mother.

They flew home that same night. Three weeks later, I received a video in the mail, of a much calmer, happier little boy (I saw him actually smiling!) with a sticky note stuck to the video that simply said, "Thank you."

The simplicity of this gift means that you can instigate this process in whatever way is appropriate. There is no official "required protocol" or methodology in application, and as such you can and should adjust to suit the environment and the needs of the person who came to you seeking balance.

In this form of healing, you should know that there is no standard set up, method or ritual. Any stagnant immovable process is restrictive, and certainly in this. Most of the time, the standard old healing room, massage table, and the basic set up are quite adequate, and appropriate for most of your clients.

Remember the Infantry catch cry? ***Improvise, Adapt and Overcome.***

Each client's body and situation will speak differently depending on what is needed and required. You as the facilitator need to be adaptable; you need to be flexible according to the changing requirements. The environment in which you heal needs to be adaptable too.

How will you handle it when a six foot paraplegic comes into see you? Will you insist he gets on the table? How about someone with severe quadriplegic spasticity? Would you demand they leave their highly supportive chair, and spasm unsecured on the table? Of course not.

No, I am not talking about moving furniture about or buying a hoist, I'm talking about adjusting you, your body and your attitude, adjusting the instrument as required for the situation.

You saw it with this sweet autistic child; he was not going to fit into the required method for healing, and any amount of logic you used to convince him that "this is how it's meant to be done", was to him just another low level noise.

If someone comes to me in a wheelchair and it's far more appropriate to leave them there, I do. I work around the chair. No amount of leather, metal, electrical current, cement, or even drugs, will interfere with the process the frequencies facilitate. I adapt so that the client's experience is all it should be. They don't come to fit into *my* comfort zone.

Back at the Children's Hospital again and Jack had just had minor surgery. I was in the waiting room, throwing anxious glances at the intercom, poised to go down to Recovery. This round had been minor: Botox injected into his calves to reduce spasticity, but still, handing your semi-conscious child over to an anaesthetist, and watching them disappear into the unknown has to be one the hardest things I have ever had to do. Not least of all because Jack doesn't react well with general anaesthetics.

On this day in that heart-wrenching moment, as I watched the anaesthetist disappearing with my boy, another little girl was rushed past me into theatre, and was, to my relief, an immediate distraction for me.

I looked at this little frail, unconscious girl as they frantically organized her for theatre. She was tiny; apparently eight or nine, she was the size of a five year old. Her little body was ravaged with cancerous cells, and the tubes and drips going in and out of her amounted to more than her entire body weight. She had tried to keep her hair long, and although most had fallen out, still she had some straggling long patches. Bizarrely, I saw strength in that. Determination.

As I turned to walk away I heard the nurses debating the value of the surgery saying she only had hours left and "Why put her through it?" I walked down the hall to the waiting area.

The intercom, through the static, intoned "Ms Hocking. Ms Hocking to Recovery please." I barrelled through the doorway and down the hall into Recovery, my eyes seeking my boy. Found him…

"Hi, J."

Sleepy eyes opened, "Hi Mum. Time to sleep. Night."

Sleepy eyes closed.

He was tachycardic (again), and he kept holding his breath (pain response), so we were in Recovery for some time.

As we waited they brought that same little girl into Recovery.

More than any other ailment, I hate seeing children with cancer. Perhaps it's due to my own experience. The thought of any child enduring such pain and desperation, bearing the burden of those who love you who are so pained by your ordeal, having to fight for the basic human right to survive…

Andrew was with us and saw me looking at her, watching the nurses trying to get a response from her. He whispered, "Jack's okay. Help that little girl."

I used my eyes. I must have looked like I was staring at her, as I did notice one nurse kept looking at me like I was being rude. But if that seemed inappropriate, then what would they have done if I had waved my hands about like a nutter?

When you work on someone you can often see, if you're

prone to visually seeing these frequencies, a peaking of frequencies off the body. I'd never seen anything like what I saw over this child. It rapidly became like a mountain of frequency where she was housed in the middle. Her entire body was ensconced within the mountain, which reached to the floor and peaked over the top of her somewhere above the ceiling, if the pattern was to be believed.

I heard the nurses say, "Oh God. She's seizing!" as they were looking at her eyes oscillating beneath her closed lids, and the movement of her head (whoops). Just as we were heading out to the ward, her parents came in. I remember their faces so vividly. Their hearts despairing, their eyes bleary with a million desolate tears spent. There really is no pain quite like that of watching your child suffer.

Four weeks later, we were back at the hospital for a post-operative check up, and we passed the same little girl in the hall. She was walking along with a nurse, holding onto her drip pole, and giggling. Her scalp was dark with a new downy growth of hair. She looked great! She was alive.

I'm neither recommending nor suggesting you step this far outside the comfort zone. I like a challenge, enjoy an adventure, but still I don't seek situations like this. However, I do respect the incidental education that I am privy to and when placed in a situation like this I do readily grasp the opportunity to learn a little more.

This is one of those situations I told you about where you may never hear a "thank you" and you may never know for sure if you assisted the healing (although it's highly likely) or if God stepped in with one of those miracles. One by one, as a facilitator in healing there will be people you assist, you initiate, who will never say thank you, or report the healing that took place, or express the joy they are now able to know. They may never in this lifetime even hear your name or see your face. And that is how it should be. That is the gift you have as a healing facilitator.

These frequencies are so subtle, and unpretentious, bound to nothing yet related to everything. *They* couldn't be more flexible. *We* are where the challenge lies.

You never know who may be watching. You never know who may be affected.

I was assisting an associate and his organization teaching at a healing workshop that was being run in my home town of Melbourne. At this workshop I experienced the very best and worst of the new age crowd. Assisting at this particular workshop turned out to be a heinously cruel, but elementary lesson for me. It forced me forward.

A lot of the people attending this workshop had come to it through me, either by contacting me, or by having seen me as a client. All had come on my endorsement, and recommendation. And this workshop had a record number of attendees; hundreds.

The people attending were extraordinary. Greeting everyone as they entered, you felt powerful in their presence and privileged to share the same space with them. You could feel that all entering would leave changed. They were ready.

Sadly, the organization that was running this workshop stuffed up spectacularly, and as such, de-edified themselves to the Australian public terribly. Participants were all charged different fees for the workshop, some were charged twice, some not at all and that really was only the very tip of the iceberg. The staff were disharmonious (I'm trying to be gracious here), the volunteers were riding the ego rollercoaster hard and fast, competing fiercely for accolades and status, and all of this was blatantly obvious to the participants. For me, it was embarrassing! Cringe worthy.

Unfortunately, it didn't stop there. Personally I took an absolute flogging from some of those who couldn't see straight for the ego was jammed so tightly up their…well, anyway. Ultimately, most damaging would be that I was so associated with such unprofessional and unethical behaviour.

Despite this crap, which never let up, I stayed. The one thing that would keep me there, come what may, and was that single moment, that beautiful moment when a person recognizes the healer within, realizes it in their own hands. They get it. They feel it in their hands, and know it in their hearts. I love that! Oh god, I love that. It is exactly what I am here for, and precisely why I love to teach. To see people, one at a time, discover the miracle within themselves!

So, regardless of the distractions, I kept my focus upon the participants. Upon the people who had trusted me.

Throughout the two days, people were getting on and off massage tables, as well as working at them. One gentleman was quite tall, and during a bathroom break approached me because a recurring lower back injury had flared up from having to lean over the tables. He asked if I would help him. At the time, everyone was returning to their seats, preparing for the upcoming lecture which was just starting, so I turned to him and said,

"Come on. I'll sit next to you for a few minutes."

The expression on his face said it all: that was not the answer he had been expecting.

We sat down at the edge of the crowd, so people could still approach me as they needed, and the lecture started. People were squatting down next to me whispering any number of issues and queries, and I continued working. After a few minutes I turned to the gentleman and said, "How is the pain?"

He sat forward. His face was prepared to grimace, but instead registered shock. "The pain is gone! It's gone. It's better."

"Great." So I excused myself, as I had to get on with "assisting".

How? Why had his pain dissipated? These frequencies don't come from my hands. They flow through me, of me, around me. It seems that I am a pretty good vehicle for this for some reason, so they flow strongly. I knew that by simply sitting next to me, this gentleman would take them on. And he did. The next morning, his back felt even better again.

Six months later, at a mentoring workshop I was teaching, I was to discover that two of those attending my workshop had witnessed me sitting next to this man. As usual, it didn't even occur to me at the time that someone would be watching me or overhear the conversation. I certainly never imagined that that moment would cause those two individuals to undergo a shift all of their own, or lead them to patiently await a place at *my* courses. One of those people, Paul, is to date one of the most gifted and generous healers I know, and one from whom I, too, have learned a lot.

That ripple effect is all powerful, and bound to bring back to you whatever you chose to put out there. Be generous people. It's to your own benefit.

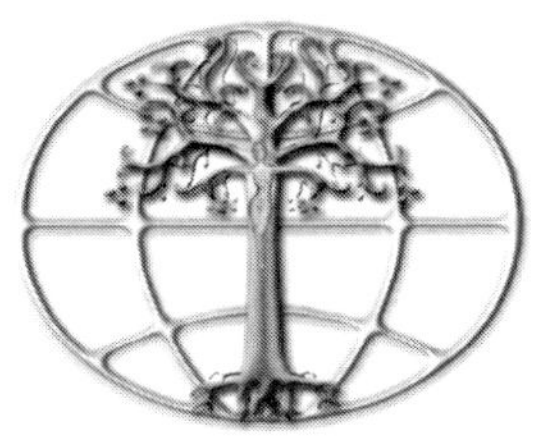

Your Journey

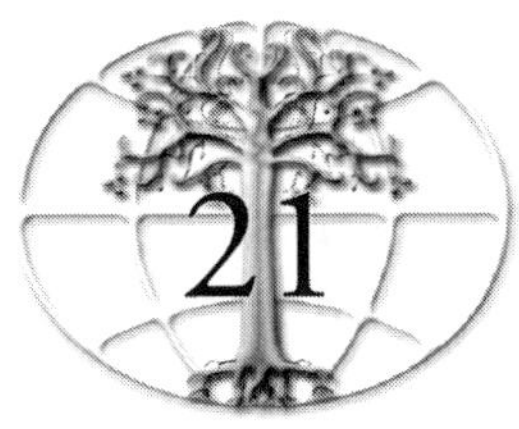

"Go cherish your soul; expel companions;
Set your habits to a life of solitude;
Then will the faculties lie fair and full within."
Ralph Waldo Emerson

Healer, heal thyself

Does it work?

The very first tumours detected were in my uterus. The treatments that combat cancer render most people infertile, and of course they had told me that there was no possibility for children. At the time it didn't worry me too much. I was nineteen or twenty, and just trying to survive. As life progressed of course, so did the ache in my heart.

Then one day I started vomiting, and it went on all day, every day. I was getting car sick, and even tram sick, smells would set me off, I would wake at 3am to vomit. I felt terrible. This went on for weeks, and I was running a personal training studio at the time. One day I was running with a client, when we ran past a café flowing with delicious aroma and I had to stop mid-run and vomit in the middle of Chapel

Street, in Melbourne. Most undignified. I could endure it no more, and went to my doctor.

It was fair enough that they assumed cancer again. With my history you would. They ran all sorts of tests, including bloods, and then I received a call to come in and get the results. As I skulked in, anticipating another death sentence, my doctor looked up at me from the file in front of her, astonishment owning her face. I took a hopeful stab,

"All clear?" I tried to avoid pleading.

"No. Pregnant."

"Who is?"

"You're pregnant." She smiled.

"Have you got the right file?" Obviously not. Surely not.

"You're pregnant, Mel."

She was serious. I was reeling. But rapidly another feeling was taking over..."Where can I vomit?" Three pregnancies later I assure you, I am the vomit master.

Recently, at a huge festival event where we had been presenting, a woman asked me how this gift in healing had affected my life. I started to go into my usual explanation of how the entire household had changed when my friend, Doug, interrupted and said, "No, Mel, *you.* Has it changed you?"

For the first time I addressed exactly how it had affected me. Physically, to look at me you would never know I have been through the health challenges that I have. In fact, most people are surprised to discover I have had three children, let alone anything like a terminal disease. If you knew what to look for there were signs that I had had a brain tumour, but gradually over the last few years even these have dissipated. I used to have one pupil larger than the other, but no longer. I had lost taste from one side of my tongue: no more. And I no longer suffer from the blinding, nauseating headache; not for three years now. The fact remains that, as I write, it is eleven years ago that they gave me two weeks to live. But even more than this… I have *three* children.

Yes, the Quantum Bioenergetic balancing technique™ works. My son, refusing healing for his physical disability, has experienced instant changes when he has asked me for them. The kids will ask if I will "zap" them, and healings occur. As a mother this is such a great gift, because if your baby is colicky, or your toddler feverish, the relief is almost instant. If your partner is arthritic, your mother-in-law is retaining fluid, your friend's heart is aching, you can offer relief. Not always, but then we've addressed that. Phenomenal stuff.

You can heal yourself.

Using these same frequencies, *you can heal yourself.*

For some of you, this is why you picked up this book. Others may not realize it, or they maybe starting to, but true healing is already occurring within, in the process of you recognizing this gift regardless of whether the lessons and "how-tos" have been tried out or not.

After we casually met at a party, a wonderful Kiwi (New Zealander) gentleman made the decision to attend one of our workshops with his wife. This gentleman was remarkably fit, having been a professional athlete for many years, and his health was excellent. He told me later that he hadn't expected any healing to occur.

Yet weeks later, he had gradually undergone an extraordinary transition in himself. He had dropped a few kilograms in weight without any real effort, he was more energized, but even more, he had noticed people seemed to be seeing him differently. New and great opportunities were being put before him, in and outside of work. These changes were distinct and palpable for him.

There is always a healing. Frequently, the healing will be what you had hoped for. However, often, in serendipity, the healing is far greater than you could ever have anticipated. A life changing experience, just for you.

The process of self healing is remarkably easy. Already

you are familiar with how to draw the frequency through your body instrumentally. You did it in lesson, as you developed your sensory awareness of it. You may or may not have worked over a body, be it the cat, a friend, your tomato plants, or a glass of water. I know, with this recognition already in place within you, that you will be amazed at how readily self healing can take place. Let's get to it…

Find a place where you are physically comfortable. You do not need to lie down, but really it is most practical for most of us to be truly relaxed. There is also the consideration that you may have large gross motor registers, so lying down can also be viewed as a safer option. Personally, if the environment is appropriate, I lie on my back as I would if I were on the table.

Close your eyes. Yes, you're allowed to close your eyes this time. However, you might want to read through the directions first.

With your eyes closed, your first directive is to utilize that subconscious servo-mechanism we mentioned earlier. Make the decision for the frequencies to flow, as clearly as mentally saying aloud "*the frequencies can now flow*". Give intent.

There is an incredibly receptive meridian point positioned in the middle of your upper lip, halfway between the base of your nose, and your actual lip line. This point is extraordinarily powerful in the transition of these frequencies, as the pericardium 8 is for recognition through the hands. Technically it's known as GC27. *Appendix 1, diagram IX.*

Now, with your eyes closed, focus your attention (or *intention*) on this point on your upper lip. Stay on that point; allow the frequencies to flow from this point. Instantly, you will feel the frequency radiate out from this point, uniformly, the sensation flowing viscous and rich like warm honey. This initial flow puts in place that constant frequency sensation familiar to you, filling you and flowing through you. It is as distinct as it is rapid, travelling down, slipping through your upper body, down your arms and into your hands (you'll feel it "kick" into your hands as it arrives). Listen to it, *feel* it as it flows right through you.

You know its flowing; you know its present… Now let go. Quiet the mind chatter; focus on the colours behind your closed lids. Let yourself just flow…

The place where you want to go is that place between awake and asleep. That gap in time where you remember all your dreams clearly. The simplest way I know to visit this point, and allow my mind to travel in depth is to "step back".

When you look into the back of your eyelids with your eyes closed, you will see colours. Moving, gliding, there are two specific colour patterns that people tend to see. One pattern starts with a mauve or purple moving then into other colour members of that group, the other initiates with red (no, not the red you see from the light glowing through your closed eyelid).

In order to step back from here, simply and consciously move backwards, away from the colour behind you eyes and into the depths of your mind. Visualize yourself actually moving backwards into your mind… the rest of this experience I will leave to you, rather than describe it and pre-empt. Physically, yes, you can focus on a specific ailment or injury whilst in a self healing state, if you want to.

Lynn, a stunning woman, is in her late fifties, but looks like she's in her mid-thirties. She tells me when she goes to bed at night she says, "Okay frequencies it is time for my face lift." She closes her eyes, and instantly feels the frequency flowing through her; her eyelids flicker and a muscle twitch here and there… And she rises the next day, stunning again. I'm afraid I can make no guarantees here.

Ultimately, as with distance healings, utterly immersing yourself in frequency as you already have will bring about whatever you require, whatever is most appropriate.

Congratulations, my friend, for you now have within you all you require to heal yourself.

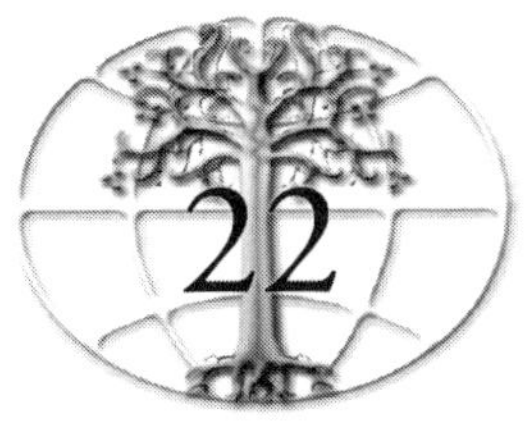

"We make a living by what we do.
We make a life by what we give."
Winston Churchill

Common Sense Practice

Rest assured, in this part of the book I'll be stating the obvious. Prepare yourself for it, because sometimes the obvious can be brutal in reminding us that we have wandered from the path a little. Sometimes we just need to hear it plainly.

A lot of the people who choose to come and learn the process of the Quantum Bioenergetic balancing technique™ will not go out and practice as a "healing facilitator". Many find they can integrate this healing ability into what they are already doing, if they already work in any area of medicine, therapy or healing generally. A lot of people come to self heal, and some occasionally work on their family or friends.

This part of the book is about conduct, be it with actual clients or just with friends or family. And it's about common sense conduct, and, in a nutshell, doing the right thing by the person entrusting themselves to you.

First of all, let's look at the environment you're inviting people into.

In order to maximize the experience for them and for you, you can put some simple yet effective factors into the environment around you both. In short: keep it simple.

My healing rooms, the actual rooms in which I do sessions, are almost "clean" rooms. They are deliberately uncluttered and uncomplicated in appearance, scents, and lighting. I have a few chairs, a desk, a few basic essentials, and yes, a treatment table: a massage table or a beautician's table – this type of table is by far the easiest to work around when implementing this process. The only difference is my study at home, where I occasionally see people; there the walls are covered in my kids' artwork wherever there are no books.

Why is the room set up like this? You don't want to interfere or take away from the client's experience. The physical stuff will take care of itself regardless, but why miss the experience if you don't have to, right? So the lighting is soft and inoffensive so they can relax. The noise is reduced to its minimum, and as I refer to it, "You may hear some domestic white noise.", but I have no relaxing music, or tinkling noises, or resonant sounds. You don't want them to miss what is being communicated to them because you cranked up your favourite Hendrix riff.

Regarding the appearance and the clutter issue, again keep it quiet. Do you recall the lady who opened her eyes and couldn't believe the wondrous geometric patterns on the ceiling? It was a plain white ceiling. Perhaps it's the influence of the autism in Jack, but it seems to be in a visually quiet room we can understand more. And in my experience, when you discuss the session with people afterwards they seem more inclined to focus and share when in a quiet environment.

There is also the issue that these frequencies get stronger with distance. You don't need to be on top of the body, in fact once you're into it, you shouldn't be right on the body at all.

I want a spacious room I can move in because distance is my ally in this. I don't need to even be facing the client to pick the frequency up through them and have them respond stronger than ever. Keep maximum space around the table, especially off the head and the feet. You'll see.

The treatment tables I use tend to be "beautician's" tables, as they have an upper body area that you can angle and elevate. This is particularly handy in the healing process, remembering of course that the client lies upon their back and access around the head is an advantage, and also great if there are blood pressure issues or postural problems. Pillows can elevate them but can get in the way, particularly during the process of Axial Initiation™. Where I can, I also get the widest table option for two reasons: we are a growing society in girth, I'm afraid, and also, it's preferable for clients to have their arms resting next to them on the table. Again, body access.

And regarding body access, I'd advise you wear no loose clothing particularly loose sleeves that may touch or distract the client. Noisy clothing isn't helpful either: cotton shirts, squeaky polyesters, and noisy jewellery can be disruptive too. Nothing worse than those clunky earrings!

Wear something you can comfortably move about in. Comfort is everything. Remember, too, that often your arms are up in the air. This raises the topic of…

Personal hygiene

Do wear deodorant. Try to avoid scents if you can, as you may recall, clients often experience scents on their journey, and you don't want to detract from their experience. If you do wear fragrance, keep it light.

Other people in the room

It is evident throughout the book that this doesn't bother me, but all the same, I wouldn't recommend it for your focus. I have nothing to hide and I'm sure you don't either, but the worried looks on the relatives' faces as the client body responds can be disconcerting. You want to keep the static in your own mind to a minimum. You've heard of "mind over matter"? This is an issue of mind over chatter; that nasty self chatter where you say things to yourself that you would never say to anyone else and it becomes louder in the face of doubting relative eyes. For the sake of the client, and your session, keep the room simple.

Ultimately, the question of whether or not someone stays in the room with them is up to the client. Naturally if it's a child, keep at least one parent handy. Same for any caregiver, related or not. A familiar face is welcome when the unfamiliar appears.

Client relations is a topic where I'm probably teaching you to suck eggs, so I will not harp on. I think "client relations" might be related to "business ethics" where you either have good people relations generally or you don't.

'The Golden Rule' is a good rule of thumb.

Professionalism. Whether or not you do this for a living is an essential; ***Discretion*** is another. People in session can have any number of responses emotionally and physically, such as crying, or calling out, channelling is another ripper, or those embarrassing bodily noises. Should any or more of these things occur during session, look upon it as an opportunity to work on your poker face, and keep going.

Above all, treat everyone with respect.

Prior Health Issues

I briefly mentioned blood pressure issues, or postural

problems before, and now I want to go into a little more detail. Do your best to address each client as their physical needs require, for example, pregnant women, people with blood pressure issues or spinal injuries, etc. But for goodness sake, don't pretend to know what you don't! People do tend to come to a "healer" expecting that you would understand what's going on with their health issue. If someone comes to me and tells me they have a disease I've never heard of before, I get terribly technical and say, "What is that?" In asking this question I am released from all pretence of being a doctor, or medical specialist.

Pregnancy alone is colourful depending on how far into the pregnancy a woman is and any particular issues she may be having. There is bound to be a lot of pillow manipulation and propping around a pregnant woman, not to mention, most will need to lie on their side while you work. In all three of my own pregnancies I vomited pretty much from conception right up to in between contractions in labour, until that baby was out. A bucket is not a bad idea too.

People know their own health problems and will know how to address what's most comfortable for themselves, so if you can accommodate it, do it. Most people lie on the table. But occasionally someone will come in with cancerous growths up their spine, or a brain tumour that dramatically alters their balance feedback, and this is when you adapt the environment for them. How? Ask them. Sometimes it's better if they sit upright. Sometimes, in the case of the brain tumour, it worked to keep the eyes open too. If you do not know the specific requirements of each client and how to adequately and safely address them, *do not pretend to*! Be honest with them. It will be better for both of you.

This brings me to the topic of medications. I have grown up in a family full of health professionals, and you know my own education, so I probably know a little more than the layman when it comes to medications. *I do not touch this.* And you shouldn't either. I advise people to keep on with their medications unless their doctor/specialist tells them otherwise. Besides anything else morally, there are legal issues at hand that you don't want to deal with.

A medical specialist, after one of his patients suffering depression had successfully weaned off her drugs after a session, sent five of his most affected patients to me for three sessions each. All of them suffered from schizophrenia and were on some fairly heavy levels of medication. I confess I was worried. I figured the last thing these people needed to hear was another voice talking to them, so I scheduled these patients when the rooms were empty of other clients. Two of the gentlemen were somewhat distressed when they first came in, however after the session, all left restful and fairly quiet. Seeing their innate calm after the session was good enough for me.

One of the gentlemen living with schizophrenia told me that during his session he had spoken to an older man, with a beard, but he knew this was not the usual people that spoke to him, so he wasn't afraid.

Weeks later, this doctor told me that all of them had had their medications reduced significantly and were doing great. You don't need to mess with medications. There are the appropriate specialists, usually those who prescribed the medications that if required, or when the need is substantiated, will do that.

Compensation for the session

Forget the whole money thing for now, and instead let's talk about *exchange*.

There are certain irrefutable laws that exist here, that cannot be messed with. The law of compensation is one of those laws. The basic law of compensation, another law based in balance, is that there must be a balance to all actions, decisions, thoughts, behaviours and even matter. The old, "what goes around comes around" is in all things true. Accept that whatever you choose to put out there (both the good and the bad) will come back upon you eventually.

In this law, the compensation or return you get for what you put out there isn't always what you may have wished or planned for. The naturally occurring balance in this, as in healing, will prioritize what is appropriate.

Occasionally, a client will come in and, if the clock permits, I will allow for the session to run overtime. I've missed many lunches doing this. It's usually because I am learning from them, or I can see we have more to learn together in the future. Invariably these people will notice we've gone over time, and amid their profuse apologies try to pay me more. I do not accept it. No doubt in exchange for my time, they gave me theirs, and a little more education along the way. I'm already well compensated from that.

In facilitating healing there does need to be an exchange. It does not have to be monetary. I've worked on a disabled child for a bag of lemons. Two people attended my course in exchange for babysitting. And like most practitioners and facilitators, I don't have the time or the energy to decipher an appropriate exchange for each individual.

So yes, I charge money. An easy and common exchange that people understand. It's also a simple way for a person to express gratitude or acknowledgement. Not everyone is comfortable vocalizing thanks. It is my choice and it is at my discretion that I charge concession rates, working on a sliding scale. A lot of the people who come to me have been chronically or seriously ill, and often off work. I can empathize with that.

Should you become, if you aren't already, a facilitator of healing, the decision is yours as to how you approach the topic of exchange. To provide any service for free, will do neither of you benefit. People will discount the amazing gift you have as "worthless", and not worth consideration, and therefore effectively minimize or refuse the healing. Their perception is important as it will affect their intention. The seeds of doubt will carry back to you. Please don't underestimate those irrefutable laws of existence on this planet.

For the Record

If you've reached this page, clearly you have read the book and know more about this process of healing than most people. Should you already be in an environment of healing professionally, the subtlety of quantum bioenergetics means you can already adapt it to your own work.

However, unless you've trained with melissa hocking healing, or with Quantum BioEnergetics International, and are accredited through us, please understand that we cannot endorse you as a facilitator of the Quantum Bioenergetic balancing technique™.

We do have register of those that have trained with us, their certification is recognized internationally, and we happily recommend any facilitator should people enquire.

Also, if you are seeking a facilitator of the Quantum Bioenergetic Balancing Technique™, or even me, please do be wary of the unqualified or unaccredited, or those who would otherwise mislead you.

Above all, never misrepresent yourself. The price you would pay could never be worth it.

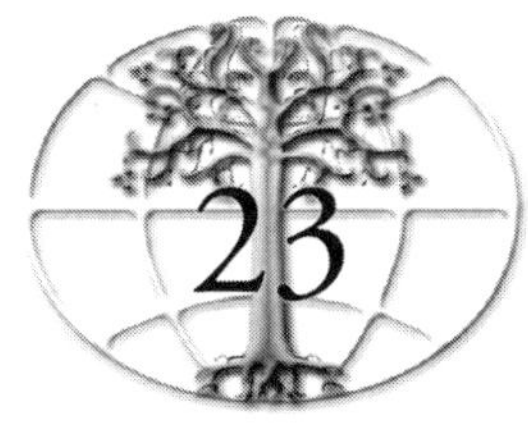

"It is our choices, far more than our abilities that determine who we are."
Professor Dumbledore
Harry Potter and the Chamber of Secrets

Additional Enhancement

Recently we launched our children's program through melissa hocking-healing. We've initiated this program through a known children's foundation in Australia. While the program is available to children affected by illness or disease, we also invite any and all children to play: typical kids, kids with disabilities, children facing any challenges and children who blissfully have none.

The kids in this program are aged between seven and eleven, and with the incredible staff, all qualified child care givers, off we go. For two hours these kids are immersed in an environment of frequency, and in that environment they work with, and are taught how to use these frequencies. You can imagine the power of placing these kids in this environment, can't you? The potential to heal is theirs. To walk away with knowledge of the power within, prior to entering a fragile and volatile adolescence, is incredible too.

In the last twenty minutes of the program I get the kids to go and get Mum, or Dad, or whoever brought them, and the kids then facilitate a session on them. Of course, these children are better facilitators than most of us! They teach me so much. The parents' faces are priceless when they enter the room and are reintroduced to the little empowered warriors they dropped off only a couple of hours ago.

At one of these programs, as they were leaving, a gorgeous little boy with leukaemia pulled on my shirt to get my attention. I squatted down to meet him. His papery, withered little hand cupped my ear as he whispered, "I always knew I was magic!"

Some weeks later this little man left us, and as his legacy this is now the name of this program;

I Always Knew I was Magic

Gliding in

When the session is finished on the table, and you have indicated so to your client, you will see some distinct changes in your client. Not least of all is the smile that comes readily to them.

There are times when the experience is huge for them, and they seem quite disoriented, having trouble focusing and listening after their session. Huge physical registers aren't always the signpost for this either. Some people may have shown next to no registers, yet they can look like this too. Please remember that the physical end of this is only a fraction of the whole.

This is another good reason for taking the time to debrief the client after their session and discuss it. Giving them the opportunity to find their feet again, you can gauge where they're at and if they need a little help to re-stabilize.

Plus you get to document and study their experience, and your own.

In the middle of a workshop, overnight, I was conducting an Axial Initiation™ on a woman that was attending the workshop as a participant. Two of her friends had watched as I put this procedure in place for her. The ladies were stunned from what we had ended up witnessing at our end. This was no small process for her and either side of it she had to spend two whole days immersed in frequency, at the workshop, as she learnt how to use it.

When she got off the table, she just wasn't here. One look into her eyes told you that. In 'normal' circumstances she would have come back in her own time, but on this occasion I knew she needed to be functional intellectually. She'd paid money for this course, and in her current euphoric, air-headedness it would have been money down the drain.

This is another of those "educational" moments, where I felt I was standing outside my body looking on, watching myself, in order to learn this. I took her hands and looked into her eyes, and knew she needed to come back a little faster. So I effectively glided her back into her body, which is not a dissimilar feeling to the dropping through your hands, using the frequencies. It feels very much like a wave gently and evenly glides through you, you actually feel people landing back "on their feet". It's very cool. The effect is immediate and it enables them to be very clear again.

Some people have referred to this as "grounding", but I personally find this inappropriate not least of all because grounding is usually used as a tool against fear. There is nothing to fear in using these frequencies. Take it from a person that has had a huge amount of experience with them. The only thing I have truly feared in this is me and my own potential inadequacies.

To me this process of gliding in is more a rebalance or a recheck. It seems to enable people to function a little more clearly at this level while whatever is occurring at a deeper or far reaching level still goes on. Experience has shown that reconnecting clarity in this way doesn't take away from the healing process. It doesn't seem to stop or disable the frequencies in any way.

When I 'glide someone in' people are able to function in their incidental existence more clearly without losing any of the experience or the healing. It's a simple tool that absolutely has its place in this, in healing. The physical healing really is the tool through which the message is carried. The physical healing is the least of it.

A genuinely gifted clairvoyant lady, after learning this technique, found it a great asset for her own clients when she completes their readings. A psychologist working with children that have suffered sexual abuse has also found it enriching for her clients.

More physical, in that you hold their hands, I don't suggest you go out there and start "gliding" people in it at work tomorrow. It could be perceived as being more intrusive, particularly as the wave-like sensation is distinct. But in its place, this is unprecedented and intense.

Resonant Entrainment

Both of the previous environments I mention, the group situation and the distance healings, demonstrate the power of entrainment.

When I've got the basics out of the way, I love to show attendees at the courses the infinite quantum element of these frequencies and how readily they flourish and create a uniform vibration.

As you discover a state of balance in a person's body, the frequencies find a common resonance or vibration. The cellular community undergoes entrainment.

In multiple bodies, you can cause the same uniformity to

occur. Some people are big physical responders, some don't respond at all. However, if I facilitate between multiple bodies, I somehow initiate a common resonance between them. All the registers not only happen at a similar level, but also usually if one has a muscular twitch through the leg, so does the other. The most bodies I've tried this with at any one time is six, and all entrained remarkably.

Every physical body you work on will feel different, because every body, human or otherwise, is unique. Yet under this common entrainment, the feel of each body is also common: the feel the same. Entertaining to watch, yes, but fascinating to explore.

Hands on

Speaking of things physical, these frequencies can be used, and quite effectively, in a hands-on technique. That very first broken foot I worked on was with this hands-on method. There is place for this technique, however I find it rarely.

For a specific injury, this is great. For localized bruises or cuts, or independent joint problems such as a sprained ankle or a "frozen" joint, this can be handy.

Lightly place your hands upon the affected area and allow the frequencies to flow through your hands. Usually there are comments from the client about how hot my hands feel within seconds. And the same rule applies: when you're "bored", finish.

Distance Healings

The phone rang. It was late in the evening, well past most civilized caller's hours, so I answered the phone knowing that the person at the other end would be anxious in some way. As I answered, sure enough, I heard the tell tale bleeps indicating that it was long distance.

An older gentleman's strained and emotional voice started begging me to help his wife. They lived in a town called McKay in Northern Queensland, about 2,500 kilometres from where I was. They had already planned a trip down to Melbourne, and were scheduled for sessions, but apparently his wife's body was operating on a different schedule. As they arrived at the airport she had suffered a heart attack.

She was rushed to the hospital, and on admission underwent, as you would, a huge array of tests. Her blood chemistry was dramatically askew, so much so that she was scheduled for a full blood transfusion early the next morning. Her prior health issues and her age suggested that this in itself was hugely risky, hence the phone call.

"Can you help her? We'll fly you up, and pay all your expenses. I can call the airline now if you like."

It was almost midnight.

"No, no. What I need to know is where you are."

He gave me the name of the hospital in McKay, and then all the details of what she looked like, what room number, the phone number in there… I interrupted.

"I need to ask you to do me a favour…"

"I'll transfer the money right now!" His voice faded a little as he moved away from the handpiece, apparently accosting a staff member saying "Is there a computer I can use?"

"No! Don't worry about that." I went on to ask him if he would stay by his wife's bedside for the next thirty minutes or so, and write down anything unusual in her reactions. I would do a distance healing. And on this occasion, as we have done several times since, I wanted to document it at their end while I worked from mine.

Distance healings are remarkably easy to conduct with this process of healing. All I needed was her name and her whereabouts in order to "send" it to her. In distance healings, I simply put myself into the state, allowing the frequencies to take hold and flow through me. And yes, I have all the registers that my body cares to (most of which I am unaware of until someone tells me about them). The difference to a self healing is that I direct the session elsewhere. I "send" it to the client. Unlike self healing, I don't fall asleep in record time, probably because I am focused on sending it to someone else.

How do I send it? Intent is the short answer. The explanation is that I utilize that same "servo-mechanism" we mentioned in instrumentally choreographing the flow of frequency more effectively or efficiently. In this, distance work, I deliberately direct the session to the client, consciously focusing only on who and where they are. No more.

I did consider, and it was suggested from one of the healers I had studied with, somehow mentally working over a body, visualizing the body and walking myself and the frequencies over it. This seemed a little silly, felt worse, and in its attempted deliberate control, was ultimately quite ineffective. Remember that "trying too hard" thing? Under such guidance for those few weeks, distance healings were disastrous.

Then I recalled that all I had to do was immerse the body within the frequencies, and between the two, the body and the frequencies, they'd work it all out. So this is what I did, from a distance, between Melbourne and McKay that night.

The gentleman to his credit did a remarkable job of note-taking, and even at one point, when the nursing staff thought his wife was seizing, told them not to touch her. He noted her eyes blinking rapidly, her breathing shuddering, but even more interesting were all the monitors she was hooked up to. Having just had a heart attack she was monitored intensely for all her blood pressure, heart rates, oxygen saturation, etc. And throughout the session, about twenty five minutes, for the first time since she was admitted her heart rate slowed and steadied, and her blood pressure also became stable. His notes also included the nurses' astonishment. Throughout the session they checked that all the monitors were connected and functioning, because they "couldn't be reading properly". The next morning her blood chemistry was normal, she no longer required transfusing, and there appeared to be no permanent damage to the heart. They were able to go home.

Again, and I really am not trying to get you to attend the courses, but it is far easier to be walked through this process live than to have it taught to you in the written word. It makes a lot more sense, and is far more readily recognized at a deeper level by you, when someone else can walk you through it for the first time. Then you can *feel* it, recognize it.

Distance healings have dramatic results. Multiple times now, we've been privileged to have someone witness the goings-on at their end, while the session is conducted. Including a time when I worked on my own father from several hundred kilometres away. The sessions are no less effective physically, so it would appear, but what I find more exciting is that a lot of these distance clients refer to the new "calm" they feel. That peace in their heart is the one thing I can assure people they will feel post session.

I have to wonder, with the dramatic nature of a distance healing, if it somehow relates to the frequencies getting stronger with distance. To refer to physical distance would be naive, given the knowledge we now share, and of course in quantum theory there is no distance! As I write there are numerous studies, findings and theories parading through my memory to explain it, from simply putting it "out there in the ether", to all things vibrating, evolving and having memory, to various vibratory theory, parallel membranes, electromagnetic calibrations, and projection of thought.

But above all I think of light, in its all encompassing presence… in the *Keys of Enoch; the Book of Knowledge*; "*Here the mind is able to go beyond the static levels (of the physical) into living divinity… (and of the healing) All there may be is a quiet super-sensitivity within the interplay of the universal mind.*"

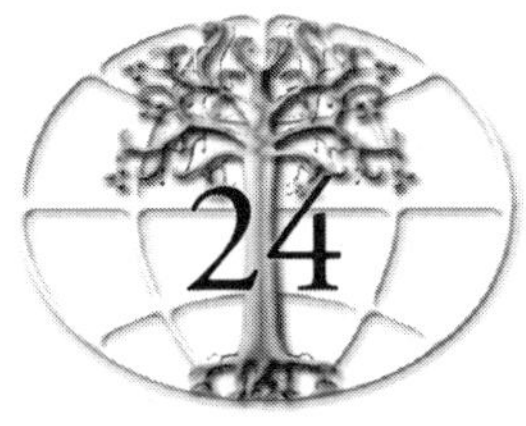

"There are two ways to live your life.
One is as though nothing is a miracle.
The other is as though everything is a miracle."
Albert Einstein

One for the Road

Y***ou are more powerful than you know***

One of the most overused graphic images we see these days is that of a single drop of water falling into a large body of still water. I know you've seen it somewhere. I refer to it as the "drop in the ocean", and not just because I think big. This is just the effect you have in your healing capacity. You see a client, help to balance them and assist them to heal themselves, and a single drop falls to the still water. The ripples start to go out… people share what they experienced, what they heard someone else experienced, what they feel in their hands because someone (you) showed them how to, and the figures grow exponentially. The majority of the people you ultimately affect, or even help to heal, may be unknown to you. And the physical healing, miraculous as it may be, will be the least of it.

Kryon uses a great analogy to describe this affect; "*Imagine walking through fertile lands for years. Everywhere you go, you plant seeds. These seeds are planted automatically, because wherever you step, your very presence leaves them. Years pass and you sit at home wondering if you've done anything at all for planet Earth. You agonize over your seeming nothingness since you never get to return to the place where you walked and take a look. If you could see it, you'd see forests and giant plants, spectacular flowering fields, all with your name on them. Such is the way it works when you're in duality.*"

Here is where I ask you to put your ego away. No-one is watching you now. Even just for the few moments it takes for you to absorb these words, for even if tomorrow your conscious memory has no recollection of what I am about to say to you, it won't matter. For your heart will. For your heart already knew this about you. You are not where you are right now, not reading this book at this very moment, by accident.

Some of the greatest healers are not, and may never be known to us. Think about it…

At this time, there is a woman clothed in the tradition of Islam, housed within a country that, as a woman, is oppressive, yet she can touch someone and change their lives. She receives no respect, and certainly no recognition. She seeks neither fortune, nor fame, no book deals, or syndicated television shows. She works in healing; true to her contract, true to herself. One at a time, she assists people, and one by one, she assists to change the world.

Is she a lesser "healer" because of the restricted life she has chosen? No. Am I a lesser healer because I shared this with you, through this book? No. Are you a lesser healer? Is whatever it is holding you back, restricting your life, reducing the capacity for you to share this and making you a lesser healer? No.

There is no man higher than I. There is no man lower

than I.

This is your gift. This is your gift for you to use as you choose to. If you choose to never tell anyone about it and just use it occasionally on your pussy cat or your vegetable garden, then that is exactly what is right for you.

You are loved by Spirit. You are loved, celebrated and revered, as much as the homeless man on the street, the man that takes position in the Oval room in the White House, as the newborn that just then entered a life in Vietnam. And this is your life, your contract. God loves you. Real God, that is. Whomever or whatever "God" is to you, it always pays to remember: Man is religious; God is love.

Not everyone is meant to be a healer. Not everyone needs to be a hero either. In fact for the vast majority of people reading this book these frequencies will prove themselves to be more of a catalyst into your purpose, and gift, than your primary role. That role does not have to be loud. It is yours, quietly, peacefully.

Of course, you can always use these frequencies for the purpose of healing, for both yourself and others. After all that is how they have initially presented themselves, and what an enormous treasure that is!

An eighty-six year old woman grows more than two inches as her scoliosis affected spine straightened out in a single session. A disabled child speaks, and says "Mum" for the very first time. A stroke victim moves his arm again. A man with a broken foot walks out unaided by crutches. People walk in with cancerous tumours, and leave without them.

If that was what all this gift was, for physical healing alone, what an exceptional gift it is. What do you think you'll do with it, now that you're reacquainted with it?

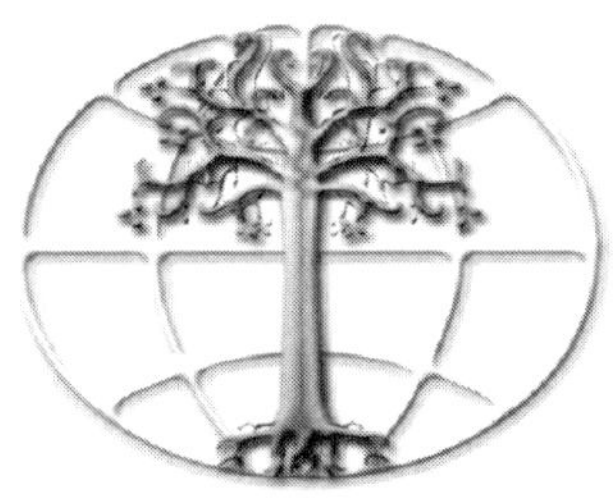

conclusion

"Well done is better than well said."
Benjamin Franklin

I was on a flight to Canberra from Melbourne which was packed to the rafters. It was a smaller plane with three seats either side of the aisle, and after being very nice to the check-in lady, I was seated on the aisle (long legs). A couple sat next to me, a man and his wife, and it was clear she was not a confident flier.

Inevitably the conversation turned to what I did for living, and I explained as much as I dared to explain to two people that had no way of getting away from me for some time. I ended up initiating the gentleman's hands, and of course, he was amazed and became very excited about it as he played with his own hands. The conversation was pleasant.

All of a sudden, a sharp pain surged through my arms, right through my index fingers and up to my shoulders. I looked down at my forearms, instinctively, to see what was happening, when BANG! The plane was hit by lightning! We were sitting just behind the wing, and I looked out to see the lightning fizzle and crackle off the tips of the wing.

The man next to me said, "How cool is that?!" It was cool.

His wife, on the other hand, became hysterical. At first it was the standard, "We're gonna die!" stuff, but then, "She did it! She did it!" She was standing up in her seat pointing at me, "She made the lightening hit us. She's got this weird electrical thing! It's her fault. Get her away from me! *Get her away from me!*"

Well, really. One stewardess was trying to calm her, another was frantically trying to persuade someone to swap seats with me (nobody wanted to sit next to Mrs. Hysteria), but worse off was her husband who just couldn't stop apologizing…to me! He would have had a few marital challenges when he got home I expect.

Every now and then I try to convince myself that this is normal. Our life hasn't become some strange adventure, and I don't have to guard my children from weirdoes (not much different from most parents actually). I try to ignore the multiple weekly offers from people who have decided I need healing because I'm possessed by the devil (actually its fatigue that has me), and I politely listen to the unsolicited readings from strangers. You do your best to ignore the defamatory crap idiots put out there, based on their own issues, and laugh off the slanderous rubbish from so-called colleagues as you pluck the daggers from your back.

But then, caught in a confined space, for a determined space in linear time, one lady goes berserk and you remember that normal isn't normal anymore.

Frequently I receive a massive thrust forward in this. Last time I experienced this, I joked that I was feeling spiritually obese, that I couldn't seem to fit back into my life anymore.

Yes, I do laugh at myself, but honestly, during such times it's still like that first rush into my life that now is. I often feel like I'm barely holding on by the tips of my fingers. You do adjust, I promise. Remember: improvise, adapt and overcome.

In the last two years particularly, it seems like time has been speeding up exponentially. There is an element of pressure for me to "get on with it", and not least of all about this book. Frequently, since I was first introduced to the fact that this is my contract, I have been taught that there is "more to follow". That's the exact phrase I know in my heart when I am told this.

Like God, or Spirit, there actually is no destination. There is no linear end to this journey, and there will always be more to follow. This journey is a staircase upward, not a doorway through which you arrive.

Take, for example, any living organism you like. You can think of any organism, for all living organisms come back to one thing: a vibration in energy. A vibration that can only exist so long as is does vibrate, and hence continually evolve.

Any real process, particularly any process that claims to work in energy healing, or human energy anatomy, is a process that demands that it, too, is enhanced and evolved. Anyone that is trying to sell you a stagnant energy process, anyone that says "this is how it's done, and that's all there is"…my advice is don't give them your credit card number.

I am constantly asked the question about whether or not people can combine or use other modalities or medical or therapeutic practices alongside the Quantum BioEnergetic balancing technique™. I am aware that people have been taught by others, others that have marketed the modality in their name, and have told people that it is the only one anyone should use. (Of course, if you use something titled by someone other than them, how will they make money off you?)

My answer to this question: Yes.

When you enter a book store, and look in the health or new age sections you will see titles on every sort of healing method, modality and belief system imaginable. Which one is the right one? They are *all* right… for someone. This gift belongs to all of us. What this gift will do, more than the physical healing, is *enhance your gift.* Be it in healing, or otherwise.

Helen's was in communication. Mine is as a Healing Facilitator/Teacher. Lynn works as a medium. How about you?

There is an amazing woman in New Zealand, Sharon, a qualified osteopath, that has learnt the ability to transfer these frequencies, and now is an even more amazing osteopath. A naturopath, Wendy, is seeing even more extraordinary healings in her clients now. A doctor, Isaac, sees a dramatic difference in his patients as they leave his consulting rooms. A nurse, Kim, working in a children's cancer ward, sees the children rest comfortably. In a country town called Kyneton, a gifted healer, Tanja, educated in multiple modalities, including this, applies whatever and all that is needed, when appropriate. When asked what technique she uses, she answers, "Intent."

I've had some serious ethical battles with myself since entering this strange healing arena. I've had the privilege of being exposed to some of the most incredibly gifted and genuine teachers and facilitators, and I've also had the misfortune of coming across some charlatans. And worst of all were the few rare individuals that had started out doing the right thing, then allowed themselves to be misled, and through ego, lost their way.

I believe in values that some seem to have forgotten like integrity, loyalty, honour, truth and love. Perhaps I am naïve because I still expect the very best of people. I expect them to do the right thing, at the very least to be honest, and unfortunately I am regularly disappointed. But I do have faith that people will see the losers for what they are. In this I have faith.

The kids and I were out in the backyard, playing on the swing set, and singing songs. As I lay on the grass in the shade, a ladybird landed on my leg.

I looked down at him. He had a broken wing. He kept flicking his little wing to straighten it out, but the transparent under wing was not retracting properly. Without thinking, I started to work on him.

He sat very still and quiet as I started to work, until I began to stretch the frequencies. It was like he was on an invisible string: my hand was about 30cm away from him, and every time I stretched the frequencies upwards, he would lift off my leg, remaining the same distance from my hand, suspended mid-air! It was really funny to watch, and the kids thought it was great; Magical Mum.

I only worked on him for a minute or two. Nearby I had a row of standard roses, and of the seven of them, only one was covered in aphids. When I finished working on him, the ladybird flew straight to that rose bush with the aphids. I stood up to look at him, and, yes, his wing was folded down perfectly. A few days later, that rose bush was completely clear of aphids. The ladybird's "thank you".

Why do people not heal?

I have had cancer and I'm still here. I have watched as others have got what would seem a lesser form of cancer, yet have declined and died so rapidly that I'm sure my mouth was still agape from the original diagnosis, when I attended the funeral.

Within a twenty-four hour period I saw my own son refused to be healed when others had seen dramatic changes in a single session. Then a man comes to me with a broken foot, and walks out, unaided, after only minutes. Why do some heal and not others?

I am not the "healer". I am an instrument through which balance and hence healing can be achieved. To paraphrase Ralph Waldo Emerson, I can take no more credit for someone's healing success, than a straw can for being hollow. And that is a great way to envision it: I am but the straw through which you drink a delicious cocktail.

Yet the question of just how responsible I am in this process will not go unchecked. I cannot bear the responsibility and take the credit for the healings, even if I wanted to, and frankly only the most delusional person would. Delusions of grandeur, that is. I do take responsibility for sharing this gift, and *how* I share this. In this I trust in integrity. It seems to me that my responsibility in this is to remain true to it. Remain in wonder and awe of it. And to respect the individuals that step through my door.

Healing takes many wondrous forms, and in this process, it is always according to what the client's body, and being, has prioritized. Some people are healed of an ailment instantly. For others it may take a few days. For some it will be a gradual unfolding, tailored for them, over a time period appropriate for them.

There is always a healing. What I cannot guarantee is that it will be what people came in hoping for.

Another exquisite element in this is that this is not maintenance therapy. When a body is exposed to these frequencies it will continue to utilize these frequencies and heal itself for as long as it needs to; sometimes in six seconds, sometimes over six months.

Why do people not heal? Only their hearts truly know the answer to that, and even then, consciously most aren't aware of that answer. For, the answer is within. For me, when people don't heal it comes down two reasons;

Intent, and whether the healing would be *Appropriate*.

All others issues or reasoning pertaining to a person not

healing fall under these two categories. Even fear.

Intent

I believe we come here, to life, in human biology, in lesson. I honestly believe there is a far greater plan than conforming to a "script"; and I am certainly not alone in this belief.

Why do some people sing legacy with their voice, while others do it just as eloquently with a paint brush?

We are each born unto this planet, without conscious memory of it, and yet with that innate knowledge of a plan or contract. I wasn't born thinking I was a healer. And yet, all roads that have placed me where I am right now have been the making of my arrival. Somehow I was born *knowing*. Everything I have done, have been and have had can be mapped to the very place I am. It has all been appropriate, including some of the more heinous experiences, because they too have given me what I needed to *recognize.*

People come to me asking to be healed. Some try to hand it to me like something in a Petri dish brought over from their doctor, something that *they* aren't willing to touch but will happily hand over to me; utterly denying the responsibility. And when I ask these same people "Are you ready to be healed?" the answer usually goes something like, "You know, I have seen everyone. I have seen Chinese herbalists, Reiki master, I've had opinion from six different specialists, and nobody is able to help me…"

The question was "Are *you* ready?" but in times like these I cannot help wondering if I should be more blunt and say "Are you responsible?"

Is the healing Appropriate?

Sometimes a healing of what they would choose isn't appropriate. It feels appropriate to me that I should win the lottery, but it too evades me. It goes against where I need to be to go forward. Perhaps there is a lesson unlearnt, or you are still amid the lesson for some reason. Several times I have stated in this book that the physical healing is the least of it. The physical ailment is usually a sign post, rather than a destination also. A disease ailment or injury can be bestowed upon you so that you may see yourself a little clearer, and know yourself a little better.

Fear falls under this title also, because in allowing fear to rule your decisions, there is usually a lesson still unfinished. And to heal prior to recognizing the lesson would be inappropriate for now.

I know some of you are still shocked from when I stated that death can sometimes be the healing. And not just for the one that dies. Regardless of how young a person is, or how they die, it was probably appropriate, for it was their life, their plan, and ultimately their choice. We are all connected. Rarely is only one person affected.

When a person comes in for session I can offer no guarantees. It's not up to me. Being a choleric individual this concept was difficult for me to adjust to early on. While I still can offer no guarantee, for I am not the healer, there is one thing all clients experience.

"*Your heart has a big ease.*" People leave the room with a new contentment within, a new quiet. People open their eyes on the table, and smile a smile that is just for them. It may not represent, and most often doesn't, a conscious awareness. Yet it is clearly present nonetheless. And not just in that instant, but in weeks, and months, even years later and remaining present in the decisions they make and how they go forward.

"*All there may be is a quiet super-sensitivity within the interplay of the universal mind.*" From *The Keys of Enoch; the Book of Knowledge.*

Thoreau once wrote that "*most men lead lives of quiet des-*

peration." I personally don't think that desperation is so quiet anymore, do you? Most people, and certainly those who seek my assistance, are seeking *relief* above all else. If all a client walked away with from a session was a heart that had eased, what a miraculous healing they had!

If we ever have the pleasure of meeting in person you will soon realize that I enjoy a good laugh. Again, another of the greater pleasures of being human, and is unique to our species, is a thoughtful sense of humour. While I laugh at myself and at the situations and circumstances of this life that have brought me to this point, please do not make the mistake of assuming I am disrespectful. I am as always, absolutely awestruck and truly humbled by the immensity of this gift bestowed upon us. I revere it as any one person should. It is divine. It's you.

I do take my work, this work, seriously. I just don't take myself that way.

You've heard of extreme sports? How about *extreme education*? If you could look up the definition of extreme education, you would find "*see* Melissa Hocking's life." Yes, my life is big, very busy, and rich with an incidental education beyond any intellectual tool we could hope to learn with. Against the instincts of the quiet, home-loving Cancerian that I am, this life forces me out the door and in front of people while the emotion in me cries "Please, no!"

As you now know, I am in a privileged, if not *very* stressful, role of parent to a "special needs" child. As such for years I have been surrounded by kids with any number, any mix, and any level of special needs. The education through this experience alone is immense. The majestic beauty of these kids…

I was in the school car park with Jack and one of his integration aides, listening as they recounted their shared day when an autistic child, Jeremy, walked over and stood next to me without looking at me, as only an autistic child would. He had often done this with me; out of nowhere he would appear, standing next to me in silence. On this day, I squatted down next to him and slowly turned my head to toward him. He turned toward me, looking down at the ground, and with a gesture I guided his eyes to meet mine.

Jeremy looked into my eyes, and I smiled gently at him. He took a deep breath and quietly said, "The noise is clearer when you're here." then turned away from me, to face forward again (the autistic version of "you're dismissed").

Life is drawing without an eraser. I choose to live it big and I choose to live it deliberately. How about you? How do you live now, with this great gift in your heart, and a newer knowledge of yourself? After all, when people see you with that small smile upon your face, they're going to wonder why it's there and they'll probably want one just like it.

Some people will think you're stupid. Some people will actually know you.

What I truly hope for is that this is simply the beginning, "the initiation" for you. I hope you step forward and learn more about you, and your journey. I don't pretend to have all the answers for you, and honestly, I doubt anyone else has them either (although there are those who will tell you *they do.* Don't give them any money!), which is why you must trust yourself first and foremost. Believe above all else, in you. I do.

In making a discovery of such magnitude as this extraordinary healing ability, it's common, perhaps even expected, that you would approach with some trepidation just how you discuss this with friends and colleagues. It's outside the square, absolutely, and by nature we would prefer to hide from it. I, too, went through this.

When a new theory arises, new and relatively untested, the first dilemma is how you will tell people about it? How do you explain to others why you have left the written script, the well-worn path laid before you? Two of our most instinctive fears as humans are the fear of rejection and the fear of criticism. To expose yourself, to your family or acquaintances with an evolved personal opinion in this way, exposes you to both these possibilities.

Know that you won't change anyone's mind. You can't. That's their job. Convincing someone, arguing your point until you're sure they are convinced, is a monumental waste of time. What is it they say? The man convinced against his will, is of the same opinion still.

Focus your energies instead on an even scarier audience; You. Letting go of rules and inset paradigms you have probably thus far lived by, that is far scarier than any friend or family member laughing in your face or making fun of you.

Beyond the possibilities of scientific hypothesis, I did have the benefit of simply feeling it in my body or between my hands. In those moments of doubt it was quite obvious that what I was feeling was true. So the niggling questions, and moments of "am I going insane?" were quelled fairly readily.

You have that ability now, too. Driving along in your car, stopped at the traffic lights, you'll find yourself playing with the frequencies between your hands. Lying in bed at night let them flow through you. You're not imagining it. They are there.

Through you, of you, within you.

Believe in you

Believe in the person you are, and the person you are about to become. Believe in the work that you do, however quietly or loudly you do it. Believe in the power within your mind, and that your heart *will* ease and sing again. Believe in the capacity of a single human to change the world for the better with a single decision. Believe, because you *can* now.

Believe in you.

So go forth Healing Facilitators! Warriors with the Light! Go forth, and be strong, knowing that every step of the way, I walk right beside you. For,

I, too, believe in you.

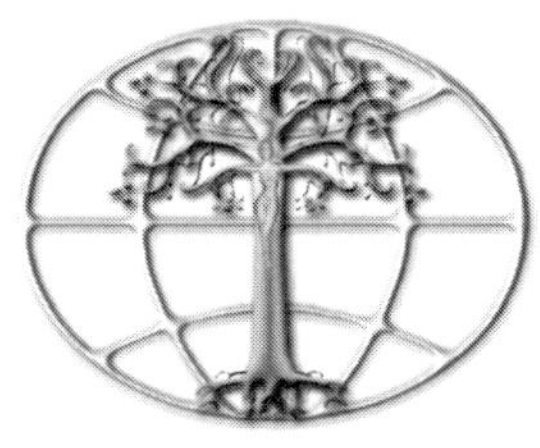

Appendices

Appendix I

Diagrams

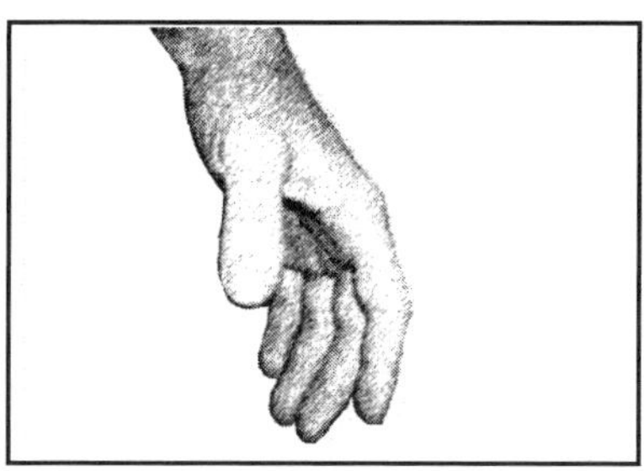

Diagram I. Normal Anatomic Position

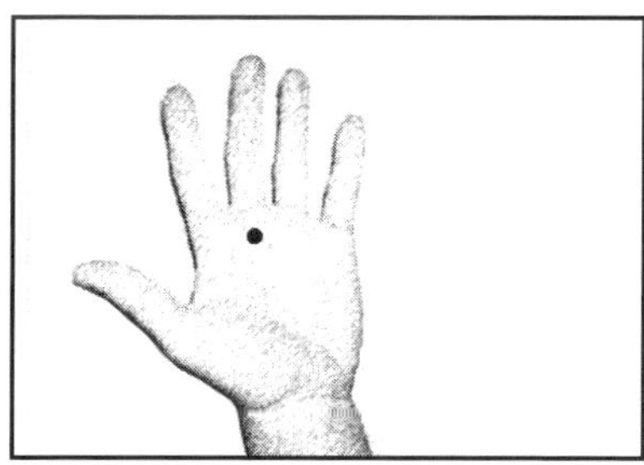

Diagram II. Pericardium 8

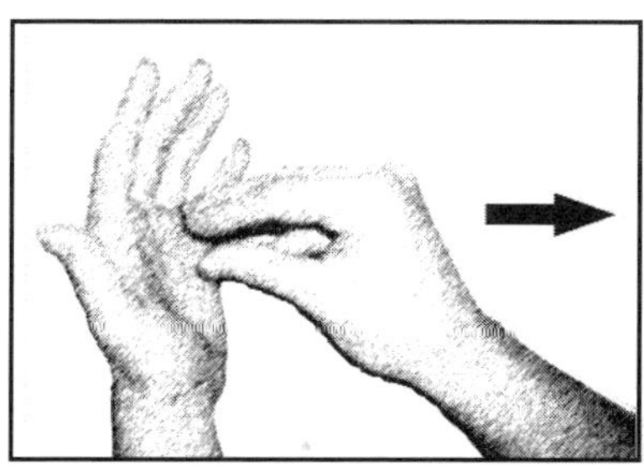

Diagram III. Pulling the Frequency Through

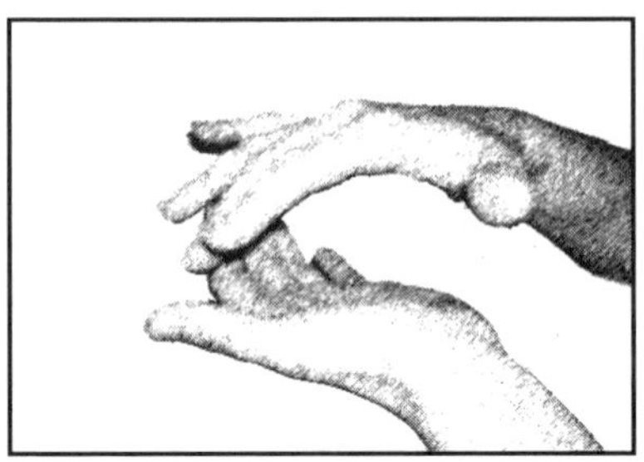

Diagram IV. Rolling the Ball

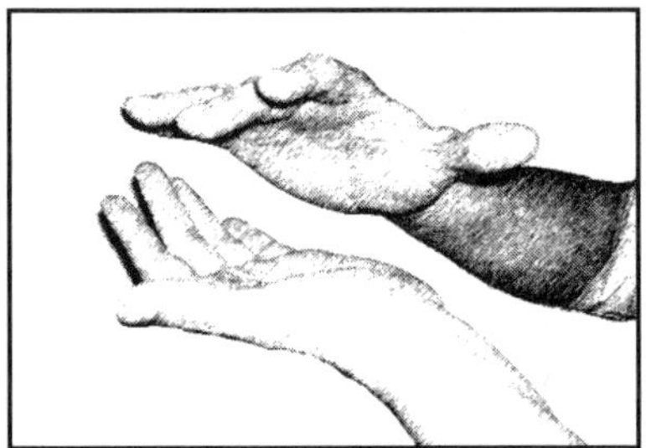

Diagram V. Snowballing – Increasing the Ball

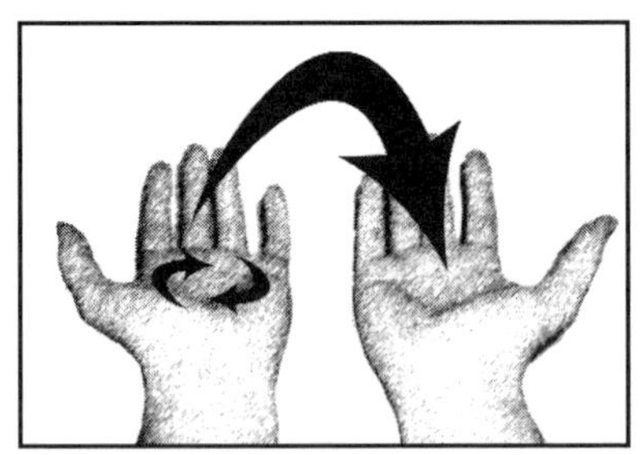

Diagram VI. Rolling Ball – Ball Toss

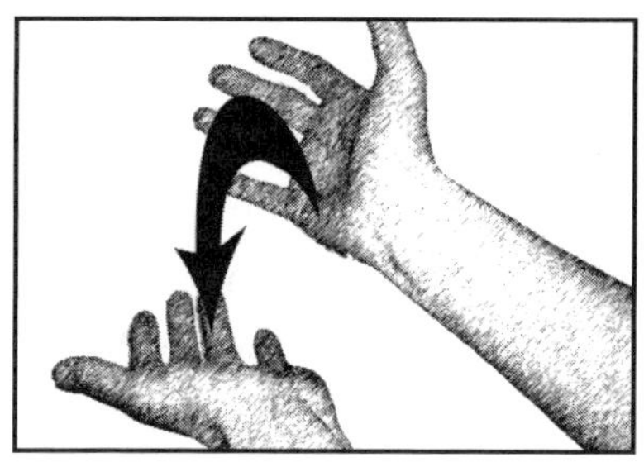

Diagram VII. Pouring the Sand

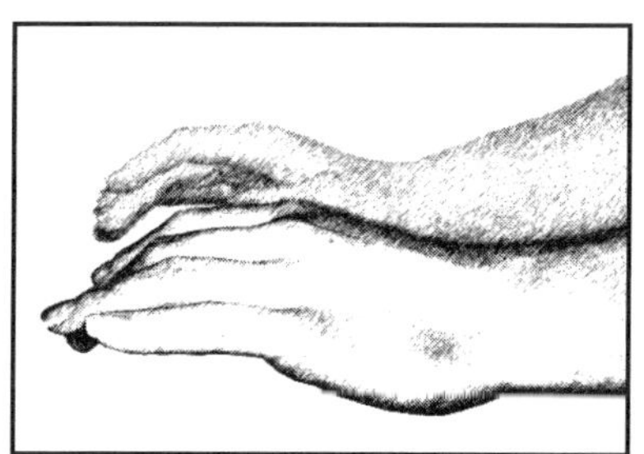

Diagram VIII. The Cushion

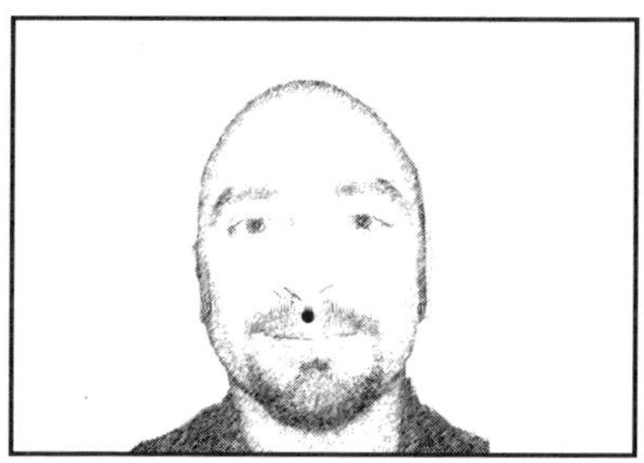

Diagram IX. GC27, Drip Placement for Self Healing

Appendix II

Definition of Terms and a few Supplementary Notes

"All Living Bodies": all known living organism; human, animal, plant, fish, water, the list goes on.

Anatomy: the science of the structure of biological organism or their parts, human, animal, plant, etc.

Axial Initiation™: This procedure, an Axial Initiation™, realigns and reconnects the communication matrix within the individual, thus re-establishing connection through the axiatonal and meridian lines of the human energy anatomy. These axiatonal lines are part of a parallel-dimensional circulatory system, connecting via the human energy anatomy that draws the basic energy for the renewal functions of the human body.

An enormous personal shift: the procedure known as an Axial Initiation™ enhances your knowledge both of yourself, and at a higher level, of the journey *you* are upon. Whatever your gift is, your purpose, your role, this procedure enhances and reacquaints you with it. For many it is the first conscious recognition of their life "contract" or purpose. A process that continues to evolve and develop, it was through this very procedure that Melissa's own healing gift was truly brought in, and enhanced.

Axiatonal lines: similar to the established acupuncture and meridian lines present in human energy anatomy, the axiatonal lines are an extension from the individual, extending and connecting outside the biological structure. Some consider these "lines" to be *higher dimensional meridians.*

Balance: the natural state of all things. To bring to or hold in equilibrium, optimal health or energy flow, resulting in a harmonious environment.

Belief: conviction of the truth or reality of a thing, based upon grounds insufficient to afford *knowledge.*

Bioacoustics: an audible resonant effect pertaining to the biology.

Bioenergetics: the study of the flow and transformation of energy/frequency in and between living organisms, and between organisms and their environment.

Biotechnology: usually refers more to the use of biological processes or living organism in technological production. An example that sadly we're all familiar with; biological weapons.

Cell: Biological: the structural unit of plant or animal life. A plant or animal structure consisting of nuclear and cytoplasmic material, enclosed by a semi-permeable membrane.

Chakra: well documented energetic vortex found within human biology. Key points readily discovered in the transference of frequency/energy during any energy work on the body. Different sources around the globe will argue the figure of how many we each have, but the general consensus is on the seven within the biological structure with more connecting through the subtle body.

Consciousness: in this volume consciousness is generally referred to as the state of being aware of one's own existence, sensations, cognitions, etc, very much in the present element.

DNA deoxyribonucleic acid: the communication foundation of human biology as we know it.

DNA Gaps: So far uncharted areas in the DNA strand as yet invisible partitions of strand yet to be identified, or understood.

DNA Helix: The double helix that is known and visible to us (actual appearance of this helix is far from orderly)

DNA Matrix: the matrix is the entire or perhaps even

"complete" structure of the DNA. As yet undetermined scientifically, it is readily speculated that there are in fact 12 strands of DNA that merge as the DNA matrix.

Energy: A little like trying to find the definition of "religion", dictionaries seem truly vague in their definition of "energy" *per se.* Generally thought of as a "force", some definitions discovered include: *a supply or source of electrical, mechanical, or other form of power, or, ability to produce action or effect.*

Energy Anatomy: refers to the "*subtle body*". Human energy anatomy is an energetic structure based within, and extending through and beyond the human biology. The energy anatomy is the connection of an individual to *all* (planet, universe, spirit, god, etc).

Entrainment: common vibration. An alignment of forces, or fields of energy, to allow maximum transfer of information or communication

Facilitation: instrumental application

Faith: belief that is not based in fact or truth.

Frequency: An all-encompassing vibratory web of communication. In general relativity the definition is; the number of cycles, oscillations or vibrations of a wave motion or an oscillation in unit time.

Healing: getting well. To restore to a state of balance, restored to health.

Healing Session: the allocated session or appointed time in which the process of healing is applied.

Human Energy Anatomy: an energetic structure based within, and extending through and extrinsic to the human biology. The energy anatomy is the connection to all in nature and beyond (planet, universe, spirit, god, etc).

Intent: the single decision to "do". Intent is the key element in instigating the process from conscious thought, to action and right through to spiritual endeavour.

Knowledge: the state of knowing; perception of fact or truth; clear and certain conscious apprehension.

Light: *(real light) the grid through which and by which all higher forms of energy are transduced so that man may receive them.*

M Theory: the collaborative mathematical theory in quantum mechanics of string theory originally discovered by Edward Wittel, co-ordinating and in the same process, discounting the apparent anomalies in multiple equations of string theory.

Physiology: the science dealing with the functioning of living organism or their parts.

Procedure: a methodical process of application. A particular course or mode of action.

Process: a continuous action, operation or series of changes taking place in a definite manner.

Quantum: Of Latin origin for the word meaning *amount.* A quantum is the smallest unit into which something can be partitioned. For example photons, the smallest known bundle of light, are the quanta of the electromagnetic field.

Quantum Bioenergetics: actually far less complex than it sounds. It is the use of quantum frequencies, via the human energy anatomy, for the purpose (in this balancing technique) of aiding the biology.

Quantum BioEnergetic Balancing technique™: This process of healing is a non-intrusive, hands-off form of healing whereby a body is safely immersed within quantum based frequencies and is then able to instigate and facilitate an appropriate healing for itself, at levels that until recent times were unbeknownst to us.

Quantum Physics (quantum mechanics): The dynamics related to atomic and subatomic systems founded in earli er discoveries of quantum theory and wave mechanics. See also *String theory.*

Quantum Theory: mathematical and scientific hypothesis and application of quantum mechanics.

Quantum Effect: almost self explanatory really. The effect of exposure, immersion or application within quantum forces/frequency. As yet immeasurable in any exacting linear measurability, and as frenetic and unpredictable as it's "source" the string.

Religion: a structured doctrine, assimilating or at least appearing to have a base in faith.

Resonance: sympathetic vibration. The excitation of an atomic or subatomic system from one energy state to another by an incident light, or an incident particle, which has exactly the requisite energy.

Spirituality: the peace and the power within you. It comes from the heart, lives within your true memory, and is all that is whole, true, and love. It's what empowers us make the hard decisions, for the greater good. It enables us to move forward when all duality of humanism cries against it. It Lives within. It resonates without.

Sonogenetically: an interesting grammatical collaboration really. Refers to the effect of sonar (a resonant tool, hence vibration) on the genetic code (DNA).

Subtle Body: see *Energy Anatomy,* Einstein is recognized to first use the term "subtle" to describe energies that were not immediately measurable by science. In reference to the body, these energies while not measurable have shown themselves present and adaptable in the human state throughout millennia.

String: The frenetic, immeasurable, unpredictable, one-dimensional subatomic particle currently thought to be the building blocks of all nature. The vibrating strand of energy within subatomic particles.

String theory: A mathematical theory that provides a unified structure to explain the properties and behaviour of elementary particles and fundamental forces, at the subatomic level. This theory is based on the string being the building block of nature, and ventures into parallel existence of planes.

Symbiosis: a relationship of mutual benefit for connected elements

Vibration: the base connection of everything in the Universe. The oscillating or periodic motion of a particle, group of particles, or solid object about its balanced state. To vibrate is to resonate. All living organism houses and is based first in a state of vibration. Hence how, in a constant state of vibration, we continue to evolve.

Zap/Zapping: the technical term given to the work Melissa does by her children, Jack, Colby and Teagan Hocking.

Appendix III

References

Amazing teachers in healing are out there for you to access. If I have resonated with you through A Healing Initiation, some of these authors may do so also.

As a Man Thinketh, by James Allen

Elegant Empowerment, Evolution of Consciousness, by Peggy Phoenix Dubro and David P. Lapierre

The God Code, The Isaiah Effect, Walking between Worlds, by Gregg Braden

The Living Energy Universe, Gary E. R. Schwartz and Linda G. S. Russek

The G.O.D Experiments, Gary E.R. Schwartz

Ageless Body, Timeless Mind: The Quantum Alternative to Growing Old, by Deepak Chopra

The *Kryon* books, from Book 1 *The End Times* to Book Ten *A New Dispensation,* Authored and channelled by Kryon and his partner Lee Carroll.

The Indigo Child, by Jan Tober and Lee Carroll

Animal Dreaming, and *Animal Messenger,* by Scott Alexander King

Quantum Touch: The Power to Heal, by Richard Gordon

A Course in Miracles, Jesus

Vibrational Medicine: Energy Healing and Spiritual Transformation, by Richard Gerber

Psycho-Cybernetics, by Maxwell Maltz

The Keys of Enoch: the Book of Knowledge, by J. J. Hurtak

Law of Success, by Napoleon Hill

Melissa Hocking

Notes

Notes

about the author

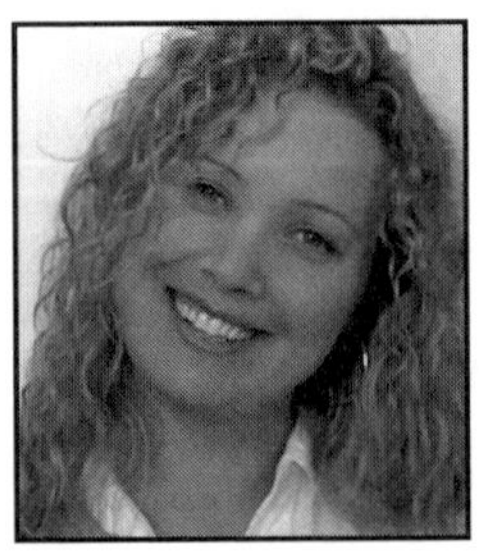

Melissa Hocking, having a double degree in Science, is an Anatomical Physiologist, and is a highly sought after speaker, teacher, and healing facilitator of Quantum BioEnergetics. The combination of Melissa's traditional education with these evolving, readily available, quantum frequencies is truly an asset. The founder of **melissa hocking healing**, co-founder of **Quantum Bioenergetics International**™, and the originator of the **Quantum Bioenergetic balancing technique**™ Melissa continues to learn and evolve alongside these amazing frequencies, her education consisting of an extraordinary convergence between the Science and the Spiritual.

For your own assurance...

The courses taught by Melissa Hocking, through Quantum BioEnergetics International, qualify and certify facilitators in the Quantum BioEnergetic balancing technique, Axial Initiation and specialised advanced level training in these areas. Presently, Melissa is the only recognised trainer of these courses. New trainers are being instructed, and in the near future, all other qualified and recognised trainers will be listed on our website, and can be verified by contacting us directly.

For your own assurance, please contact us at info@quantumbioenergetic.com to verify that your facilitator is qualified, and not misrepresenting themselves should you have any doubts.

Contact Information for Melissa Hocking

Melissa Hocking
c/- Brolga Publishing Pty Ltd
PO Box 12544
A'Beckett Street, Melbourne, Victoria
Australia, 8006
W: www.melissahocking.com E: info@melissahocking.com

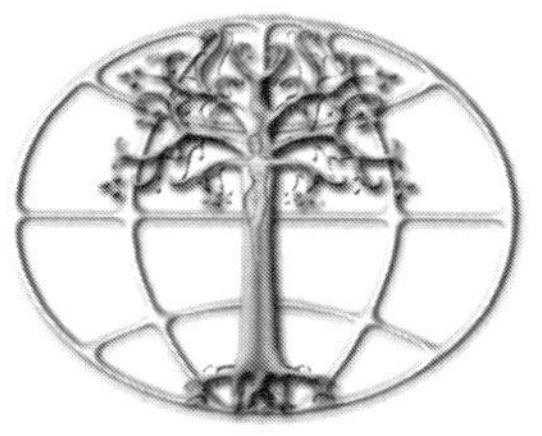

melissa hocking healing
the home of
Quantum BioEnergetics International™

We invite you to experience Healing as never before,
Immersed within the
Quantum BioEnergetic balancing technique™

To ***attend*** Melissa's courses through Quantum Bioenergetics International, or to ***co-sponsor*** a course in your area, go to
www.melissahocking.com
or email us at **info@melissahocking.com**

For further information or if seeking a qualified facilitator of Quantum Bioenergetics, please contact us directly through
www.quantumbioenergetic.com

Schedule your private session at our healing centre
melissa hocking healing
A Centre for your Health and Wellbeing
Melbourne, Australia

Order your copy of:

A Healing Initiation

Qty

ISBN 1 920785 96 5 RRP AU$24.95 .....

Postage AU$ 9.00 .....
within Aust.

____

TOTAL* $ _______

*All prices include GST

Name: ____________________

Address: ____________________

____

____

Phone: ____________________

Email address: ____________________

Method of Payment:

❑ Money Order ❑ Cheque ❑ Bankcard
❑ Mastercard ❑Visa ❑American Express

Cardholders Name: ____________________

Credit Card Number: ____________________

Signature: ____________________ Expiry Date: ________

Please allow 21 days for delivery.

Payment to:

The Better Bookshop (ABN 12 067 257 390)
PO Box 12544
A'Beckett Street, Melbourne,8006
Victoria, Australia
Fax: +61 3 9662 2622
Email: sales@brolgapublishing.com.au
Web: www.brolgapublishing.com.au